ESSENTIALS for THE CLINICAL NURSE LEADER

Janice Wilcox, DNP, RN, CNL, is assistant professor of clinical practice and director of the Clinical Nurse Leader graduate specialty at The Ohio State University College of Nursing. She has overseen the Clinical Nurse Leader Specialty since 2013 and continuously advocates for infusion of the clinical nurse leader (CNL) role in healthcare settings. Dr. Wilcox has nearly 40 years of nursing experience in a variety of acute, chronic, and home care settings and holds a joint position with The Ohio State University Wexner Medical Center/James Comprehensive Cancer Center, where she serves as a member of the Nursing Education Department, overseeing student nurse experiences and assisting with continuing education programs for nurses.

She has over 13 years of experience in nursing education, teaching at various levels of nursing with special interest in interprofessional education. Dr. Wilcox has been involved with interprofessional simulation education and has published articles and spoken at over 25 state, national, and international conferences on the importance of interprofessional simulation as a means of enhancing communication and coordination of care to ultimately improve patient outcomes. She has also contributed to three editions of the textbook *LeMone and Burke's Medical-Surgical Nursing: Clinical Reasoning in Patient Care.*

Ann Deerhake, DNP, RN, CNL, CCRN, is assistant professor of clinical practice at The Ohio State University College of Nursing. She has been an instructor within the Clinical Nurse Leader Specialty since 2011 and also teaches online in the undergraduate, RN-BSN, and graduate programs. Dr. Deerhake has worked within the CNL role for 5 years at a level 2 trauma ICU in Ohio and has nearly 30 years of nursing experience in critical care, primarily in the medical–surgical, trauma, and cardiovascular ICU. She also worked as a bedside clinical educator for more than 150 staff nurses as well as a pediatric homecare nurse for acutely ill children.

As a clinical nurse leader (CNL), Dr. Deerhake led quality improvement, clinical education, and staff development within an 18-bed ICU and 13-bed cardiovascular intensive care unit (CVICU)/progressive care unit (PCU). She and her transdisciplinary team reduced pressure ulcer rates to zero, developed and delivered annual competency education to more than 100 nurses, and assisted the ICU staff to an 84% clinical ladder promotion rate. Dr. Deerhake has been a member of the Clinical Nurse Leader Association (CNLA), CNL job analysis committee, and CNC CNL marketing committee, serving as chair. Dr. Deerhake has presented on several occasions regarding the CNL role and its impact on healthcare. Her primary area of interest is in intradisciplinary nursing communication within the critical care environment.

OTHER *ESSENTIALS* BOOKS

Essentials for the NEW NURSE PRACTITIONER: What You Really Need to Know in a Nutshell (*Aktan*)

Essentials for the A&E NURSE: Emergency Department Orientation in a Nutshell (*Buettner*)

Essentials About GI AND LIVER DISEASES FOR NURSES: What APRNs Need to Know in a Nutshell (*Chaney*)

Essentials on COMBATTING NURSE BULLYING, INCIVILITY, AND WORKPLACE VIOLENCE: What Nurses Need to Know in a Nutshell (*Ciocco*)

Essentials for the THEATRE NURSE: An Orientation and Care Guide in a Nutshell (*Criscitelli*)

Essentials for the NEONATAL NURSE: A Nursing Orientation and Care Guide in a Nutshell (*Davidson*)

Essentials for the LONG-TERM CARE NURSE: What Nursing Home and Assisted Living Nurses Need to Know in a Nutshell (*Eliopoulos*)

Essentials for the CLINICAL NURSE MANAGER: Managing a Changing Workplace in a Nutshell (*Fry*)

Essentials for Nurses About HOME INFUSION THERAPY: The Expert's Best Practice Guide in a Nutshell (*Gorski*)

Essentials for MIDWIVES: Labour & Delivery Orientation in a Nutshell (*Groll*)

Essentials for the RADIOLOGY NURSE: An Orientation and Nursing Care Guide in a Nutshell (*Grossman*)

Essentials for the CARDIAC SURGERY NURSE: Caring for Cardiac Surgery Patients in a Nutshell (*Hodge*)

Essentials for DEMENTIA CARE: What Nurses Need to Know in a Nutshell (*Miller*)

Essentials for STROKE CARE NURSING: An Expert Guide in a Nutshell (*Morrison*)

Essentials for the PAEDIATRIC NURSE: An Orientation Guide in a Nutshell (*Rupert, Young*)

Essentials for the HOSPICE NURSE: A Concise Guide to End-of-Life Care (*Wright*)

Essentials About PTSD: A Guide for Nurses and Other Health Care Professionals (*Adams*)

Essentials for the CLINICAL NURSING INSTRUCTOR: Clinical Teaching in a Nutshell (*Kan, Stabler-Haas*)

Essentials for MANAGING PATIENTS WITH A PSYCHIATRIC DISORDER: What RNs, NPs, and New Psych Nurses Need to Know (*Marshall*)

Essentials About the GYNAECOLOGIC EXAM: A Professional Guide for NPs, PAs, and Midwives (*Secor, Fantasia*)

Essentials for the CRITICAL CARE NURSE (*Landrum*)

Essentials of PRESSURE ULCER CARE FOR NURSES: How to Prevent, Detect, and Resolve Them (*Dziedzic*)

Essentials for HEALTH PROMOTION IN NURSING: Promoting Wellness (*Miller*)

Essentials of ADOLESCENT HEALTH FOR NURSING AND HEALTH PROFESSIONALS: A Care Guide (*Herrman*)

Essentials of EKGs FOR NURSES: The Rules of Identifying (*Landrum*)

Essentials for CURRICULUM DEVELOPMENT IN NURSING: How to Develop & Evaluate Educational Programmes (*McCoy*)

Essentials for the TRIAGE NURSE: An Orientation and Care Guide, Second Edition (*Visser, Montejano*)

Essentials for EVIDENCE-BASED PRACTICE in Nursing, Second Edition (*Godshall*)

Essentials for the NURSE PSYCHOTHERAPIST: The Process of Becoming (*Jones, Tusaie*)

Essentials for the CRITICAL CARE NURSE (*Hewett*)

Essentials in HEALTH INFORMATICS FOR NURSES (*Hardy*)

Essentials for the SCHOOL NURSE: What You Need to Know (*Loschiavo*)

Essentials for the CLINICAL NURSE LEADER (*Wilcox/Deerhake*)

ESSENTIALS for
THE CLINICAL NURSE LEADER

Janice Wilcox, DNP, RN, CNL
Ann Deerhake, DNP, RN, CNL, CCRN

SPRINGER PUBLISHING COMPANY

Copyright © 2021 Springer Publishing Company, LLC

All rights reserved.

No part of this publication may be reproduced, stored in a retrieval system, or transmitted in any form or by any means, electronic, mechanical, photocopying, recording, or otherwise, without the prior permission of Springer Publishing Company, LLC, or authorization through payment of the appropriate fees to the Copyright Clearance Center, Inc., 222 Rosewood Drive, Danvers, MA 01923, 978-750-8400, fax 978-646-8600, info@copyright.com or on the Web at www.copyright.com.

Springer Publishing Company, LLC
11 West 42nd Street, New York, NY 10036
www.springerpub.com
connect.springerpub.com/

Acquisitions Editor: Joseph Morita
Compositor: Amnet Systems

ISBN: 978-0-8261-6278-6

DOI: 10.1891/9780826174116

20 21 22 23 / 5 4 3 2 1

The author and the publisher of this Work have made every effort to use sources believed to be reliable to provide information that is accurate and compatible with the standards generally accepted at the time of publication. The author and publisher shall not be liable for any special, consequential, or exemplary damages resulting, in whole or in part, from the readers' use of, or reliance on, the information contained in this book. The publisher has no responsibility for the persistence or accuracy of URLs for external or third-party Internet websites referred to in this publication and does not guarantee that any content on such websites is, or will remain, accurate or appropriate.

> Contact us to receive discount rates on bulk purchases.
> We can also customize our books to meet your needs.
> For more information please contact: sales@springerpub.com

Janice Wilcox: https://orcid.org/0000-0002-7733-6843
Ann Deerhake: https://orcid.org/0000-0001-6778-6130

Publisher's Note: New and used products purchased from third-party sellers are not guaranteed for quality, authenticity, or access to any included digital components.

The ESSENTIALS series was published in the United States as the FAST FACTS series.

Contents

Preface ix
Acknowledgments xi

1. **Marketing Yourself as a Clinical Nurse Leader** 1
   Janice Wilcox

2. **Integration Into Clinical Nurse Leader Practice: Preparing to Lead** 17
   Ann Deerhake

3. **Leadership Within a Complex Environment** 35
   Janice Wilcox

4. **Microsystem Assessment and the 5Ps** 51
   Ann Deerhake

5. **Utilizing Evidence to Improve Practice** 79
   Janice Wilcox

6. **Utilizing Data and Quality Improvement Principles** 103
   Janice Wilcox

7. **Coordination of Care** 121
   Janice Wilcox

8. **Effective Change Management** 139
   Ann Deerhake

9. **Advocacy for Nursing and Populations** 157
   Ann Deerhake

10. **Disseminating Accomplishments** 173
    Janice Wilcox

Index *199*

Preface

The clinical nurse leader (CNL) is considered a valued nursing leader within healthcare and has improved care in many different organizations and healthcare settings. Even though the CNL nursing specialty was initiated nearly 20 years ago and has been shown to improve care processes, implementation within healthcare organizations has been slow and inconsistent. Many organizations have adopted this role and have done a wonderful job transitioning the newly certified CNL into practice. However, some CNLs begin their advanced nursing career initiating their positions within organizations, learning their role as they go. Other CNLs are thrust into positions that provide little orientation or onboarding, which also requires on-the-job learning.

The CNL is considered an advanced generalist and is expected to know and understand a wide variety of topics and concepts. They must be able to assess and evaluate processes, develop quality initiatives to improve practice, use evidence-based practice methodologies, communicate effectively as they collaborate with interdisciplinary teams, and be guardian of the nursing profession advocating for nursing, all while being the advanced clinician advocating for patients within their microsystem. Today's CNLs are the pioneers working to move their careers and healthcare forward while paving the way for future CNLs. This is not an easy task and is the reason this book was written. This book was written as a resource for all the practicing CNLs working hard to impact outcomes yet have little in the way of resources to assist them as they begin and continue their careers. It is difficult to remember everything that is learned in an academic program, and there is not always time to look through multiple books to find the information you need on a particular topic.

The authors of this book are both point-of-care CNLs who are continuously advocating for this very important role. They understand the pressures and constraints placed upon nursing and especially the CNL, and they understand not only the value of CNLs but also the need to justify the CNL role and positions within organizations. Practicing CNLs must understand that healthcare organizations are under financial pressures, which makes it imperative that they produce positive outcomes. The authors have compiled information on topics that are the most frequently used and often misunderstood by CNLs, as a means to assist in producing those necessary outcomes that will sustain this very important nursing role.

There are currently no other resources for CNLs. There are textbooks that help students learn the role, but nothing to help practicing CNLs, until now. This book will help you market yourself to obtain that dream position following graduation, it will provide insight into transitioning into your new CNL role, it will assist you in reviewing leadership skills to deal with the laggards during change initiatives, and it will provide you the basics of quality improvement and evidence-based practice to create projects that will move your microsystem toward positive change and allow you to be seen as the leader you were meant to be. There are also resources that will guide you in disseminating your accomplishments to organizational leaders, other CNLs, and the world. This book is a must to move the CNL movement forward.

Janice Wilcox
Ann Deerhake

Acknowledgments

We would like to acknowledge and thank all the dedicated CNLs who work tirelessly at the point of care improving patient outcomes while creating better healthcare systems. No matter what environment in which CNLs work, their efforts are invaluable to not only patients but every other discipline with which they come in contact by coordinating care services and utilizing their knowledge of systems, change, and leadership. Today's CNLs are the pioneers moving their role forward and exemplifying nursing's ability in creating better healthcare systems.

We would also like to acknowledge our families, friends, and colleagues who offered guidance and support through this project.

1

Marketing Yourself as a Clinical Nurse Leader

Janice Wilcox

"Your value doesn't decrease based on someone's inability to see your worth; enlighten them anyway!"

~Unknown

INTRODUCTION

The clinical nurse leader (CNL) nursing specialty was developed to address deficiencies and gaps in care related to quality and safety within our healthcare systems. The American Association of Colleges of Nursing (AACN; 2018a) defines the CNL as follows:

> *A master's educated nurse, prepared for practice across the continuum of care within any healthcare setting in today's changing healthcare environment. CNLs oversee care coordination, provide direct patient care in complex situations, put evidence-based practice into action, ensure patients benefit from the latest innovations in care delivery, evaluate patient outcomes and assess cohort risk and have the decision-making authority to change care plans when necessary. The CNL is a leader and active member of the interdisciplinary*

healthcare team. The implementation of the CNL role will vary across health care settings. (para. 6)

You most likely learned in your educational programs that leaders from education and practice came together to envision and initiate this new nursing role to enhance safety and improve outcomes through lateral integration of care. This lateral integration of care improves communication and practice among interprofessional teams. You have learned how to manage teams, improve processes, and initiate and sustain change through the use of evidence-based practices and the use of quality improvement tools. Your education also provided you with knowledge and skills to move care to higher standards, and you are ready to reach your goals to create change. However, obtaining your dream position may take a little work. The CNL role is relatively new, and not every organization has adopted it within its care models; therefore, marketing yourself is of great importance. This chapter provides you with tips and tools to market yourself as a CNL, obtain your dream position, and also change healthcare for the better.

After reading this chapter, you will be able to:

1. Identify strategies to guide you in creating or obtaining a CNL position
2. Recognize important steps in preparing an impactful presentation
3. Differentiate your role from other nursing leaders' roles
4. Understand the importance of maintaining a portfolio
5. Utilize available career resources

RATIONALE FOR THE CNL POSITION

When thinking about how to go about obtaining a CNL position, it is good to review and keep in mind why this first new nursing role in over 30 years was developed. A review of the facts will act as a refresher to ultimately help in marketing yourself. You probably recall the Institute of Medicine's (IOM) landmark reports from 1999 and 2000. These reports highlighted concerns within our healthcare system related to errors and gaps in care contributing to thousands of deaths per year from medical errors and safety issues. They also reported on inefficient practices with poor utilization of resources that contributed to less-than-desirable outcomes and rising healthcare costs (IOM, 1999, 2000).

This information initiated discussions regarding nursing's role in dealing with these issues. It was determined that nurses were key players in improving care and care outcomes due to their direct relationship with patients, family, and providers of care. Nurses are responsible for the development, implementation, and evaluation of care; therefore, their insight and input is invaluable in improving care. However, it was also determined that a different nurse was needed, one with a higher level of education, who would not only be the clinical expert but also be the leader at the point of care who understands systems and processes that impact care. The AACN, healthcare leaders, and educators used the information and foresight in developing the new nursing role, or the CNL (AACN, 2007).

Unfortunately, the overall healthcare system has not seen improvements in care and outcomes since the original reports were published. Sternberg (2016) reported that medical errors are now the third leading cause of death with 250,000 deaths per year, and Makary and Daniel (2016) wrote in the *BMJ* that the estimated deaths caused from medical errors in the United States to be anywhere from 200,000 to 400,000 per year. These numbers only emphasize the need for greater numbers of CNLs within healthcare organizations and will help you in marketing yourself as a CNL.

Since the initiation of the role in 2005, approximately 5,000 nurses have earned the CNL certification (Commission on Nurse Certification [CNC], 2017). Evidence is mounting on the benefits that CNLs bring to organizations. Some of the benefits seen from these nurses include decreasing readmission rates, improving incidences of patient falls and hospital-acquired infections, improving patient satisfaction scores, reducing canceled procedures, and improving nurse turnover rates (Bender, 2014; Hix, McKeon, & Walters, 2009; Moore, 2013; Sotomayor & Rankin, 2017). This is just a sampling of the benefits to organizations that you can use as starting points to develop your marketing campaign to acquire your dream position.

WHERE ARE CNLs EMPLOYED

According to the CNC (2017), data gathered from polling of current CNLs indicate the majority of CNLs work in urban acute care settings. Many organizations throughout the United States are adopting the CNL role within their microsystems with positive results. For example, the Veterans Administration (VA) was one of the first adopters of this role and continues to expand the CNL role within its organizations (U.S. Department of Veterans Affairs, n.d.). WellStar

Health System also employs many CNLs with similar results as the VA (Case-Wirth, 2018). Organizational adoption of the CNL role is expanding throughout the country with many other organizations initiating this role, but like any change process, advancement is slow.

There are other areas of nursing where you can utilize your education and skills. These include schools of nursing, where CNLs can apply their knowledge and clinical expert skills as clinical faculty teaching nursing students. Outpatient clinics, physician's practices, and home healthcare suit the CNL skill set in the way of care coordination and outcomes manager assisting the navigation of patients throughout different healthcare settings. Public health departments employ CNLs in focusing on population-wide efforts to reduce disparities in care or improve access to care of at-risk populations. Rankin, Ralyea, and Sotomayor (2017) discuss how the CNLs employed within a certain medical center collaboratively work with high-risk obstetric patients in both the acute and community settings. CNLs in both outpatient and inpatient units work collaboratively to meet the needs of these patients, ensuring they receive the screenings and care that will prevent further admissions and complications of pregnancy. CNLs can also be found working in staff development and case management positions, so your options for employment are many. As an advanced generalist, the CNL has the knowledge and skills to impact many different areas of patient care.

Initiating the Role

At times, a nurse may wish to work within an organization that does not employ CNLs as the role was envisioned, or the particular unit does not have a CNL position within the care team. This may require effort to initiate the role. Many CNLs have gained their positions from advocating for the role and themselves. Having discussions with nurse managers, nurse educators, or nursing supervisors is a good way to launch this endeavor. Make sure to meet with persons when they have time to discuss ideas and when they are not distracted with other concerns; timing can be a critical factor in presenting new initiatives. Arrange a set appointment time to meet, and then organize your thoughts and ideas to ensure you are able to get your points across in that set amount of time. Begin by discussing issues that are occurring within the unit, and explain how a certified CNL can address these issues. Keep in mind the previous information regarding the rationale for the CNL role. Healthcare leaders are absorbed with the task of improving care outcomes and quality; therefore, it is best to focus on how improvements can be achieved in any of these areas.

Essential Facts

Advocating for the initiation of your CNL role within a particular setting is critical. Presenting decision-makers with a clear picture of what you have done and/or can do clinically and financially for their organization is key!

MAKING YOUR CASE

In preparing the proposal, it is very important to also prepare the manner in which it will be delivered. Studies in neuroscience and communication are discovering that many brain processes are involved with decision-making, especially financial decision-making, and ultimately, initiation of a CNL position will impact organizations financially (Lahmiri, 2016). Your goal is to persuade others to believe that the CNL role will positively impact the unit and the organization by demonstrating the value. At the same time, from the moment you begin speaking, you are attempting to motivate and instill passion for change in those who are listening. This means you must create a sense of urgency without instilling a sense of danger. In neuroscience language, you must reach the neocortex of the brain, and to get to the neocortex, you must pass through the amygdala. Ousdal et al. (2014) state that the brain's amygdala works to avoid unpleasant or harmful events. Therefore, if the receiving message is too boring, is uninspiring, or creates a sense of threat, the amygdala (which is the flight or fight area of the brain) will inhibit the message from getting to the neocortex where the person can process it.

The "Why"

Sinek (2009, 2014) uses neuroscience philosophies in describing how to motivate and inspire when communicating by stating the "why" or your purpose or your mission prior to describing the "how" and "what" of your proposal. To determine your "why," begin with the current outcomes within the microsystem that you want to address. What are the metrics indicating in the way of quality and safety outcomes, such as falls, central line and urinary catheter infections, and pressure ulcers? What are the patient and staff satisfaction rates? What effects are the metrics having within your organization financially? These metrics will give you the "why" of your proposal.

For example, your nurse engagement rates are declining, and your unit is seeing an increase in nurse burnout and higher turnover rates. Falls rates have increased from three to seven in the past quarter, which may be contributing to the poor patient satisfaction scores and higher costs due to unreimbursed injury. These metrics will give you the "why" of your proposal. Your "why" message to the leaders may be something like "Our mission is to improve the health of those we serve and the unit is seeing an increase in falls in the last two quarters which is contributing to less than desirable patient and financial outcomes. There is also a problem with nurse engagement as the nurse turnover rate has increased dramatically over the last year. These factors are contributing to poor patient outcomes, increased financial loss for the unit and not contributing to our mission. A CNL can improve nurse retention by being a resource and mentor for newer staff members, coordinate and oversee care to address why patients are falling, and ensure the processes are in place to maintain safety efforts in decreasing falls, which will ultimately improve patient and financial unit outcomes" (Sinek 2014). In describing your cause in this manner, you are able to create a sense of urgency or a "need" that these issues must be addressed promptly, without losing the attention of those who are listening. Viewing Sinek's (2014) YouTube video may provide insight into creating a talk that will achieve the results you desire.

The "How"

Your "how" is actually how you are going to improve the problems on your unit. When explaining how you are going to improve processes, you may want to bring in the roles of the CNL. Managers and administrators do not always understand the CNL; therefore, you may need to explain how the role improves care and processes. Use your knowledge of evidence-based practice to demonstrate the value of the CNL. Obtain literature that compares CNL outcomes on similar units. As an example, Ott et al. (2009) discuss the value of the CNL to the VA in reducing readmissions of heart failure patients. A CNL wishing to work on an inpatient heart failure unit can use this evidence to back the claims of the benefits that the role will bring to the unit.

It may be helpful to gather several pieces of literature to back your claims, and it is not always necessary to have the evidence from your particular specialty area, but it may be helpful as long as you have evidence of success. Highlight the evidence and illustrate the value that you will bring by outlining what you will do to achieve the outcomes. Following are examples based on each CNL role; however, you will want to combine this information into a concise illustration of how you will go about improving care and processes as you may not have time to address each of these roles individually in your presentation. Consider the timeframe you will have, and prepare your talk to highlight the most relevant points to your particular situation. Refer to Table 1.1 for a complete list of the different AACN CNL roles.

In addressing the common battle of patient adherence to treatment plans and readmissions, which contribute to declining patient conditions and financial losses for the organization, the CNL may choose to describe their contributions as follows:

- **Clinician:** Using expertise in the area of heart failure and knowledge of the best evidence in caring for heart failure patients, the CNL provides and evaluates care to ensure positive outcomes by rounding daily on patients; recognizes changes in conditions that require immediate attention; communicates promptly to the interprofessional team ensuring timely interventions; acts as a staff resource in planning and coordinating care, which is patient centered including family and community.
- **Outcomes manager:** Shares outcomes of care with interprofessional teams to strategize ways of improving care; implements attainable patient discharge goals and maintains contact with the patient/family post discharge to identify early changes in condition and prevention of hospital readmissions; alerts care team of changes in order to address patient changes in condition promptly.
- **Client advocate:** Acts as a communication conduit between the patient and the interprofessional team while empowering the patient to be a voice in their treatment plan; provides explanations and answers to the patient/family on different types of therapies, treatments, procedures, and medications; confers with social workers and case managers to ensure available financial resources for treatments and medications.
- **Educator:** Educates patients and families on the stages, signs, and symptoms of heart failure to ensure understanding of what to expect and when to call providers; reviews medications and the importance of adhering to medication schedules and revises schedules to meet the individual patient needs; creates a step-by-step daily plan for each patient based upon their particular individual needs.
- **Information manager:** Reviews documentation to ensure provision of care is complete and that documentation reflects what actually occurred; relays information to staff regarding latest heart failure treatments and technologies; measures and critiques

Table 1.1

American Association of Colleges of Nursing (AACN) Clinical Nurse Leader Roles

Clinician	Designer/coordinator/integrator/evaluator of care to individuals, families, groups, communities, and populations; able to understand the rationale for care and competently deliver this care to an increasingly complex and diverse population in multiple environments. The CNL provides care at the point of care to individuals across the life span with particular emphasis on health promotion and risk reduction services.
Outcomes manager	Synthesizes data, information, and knowledge to evaluate and achieve optimal client outcomes.
Client advocate	Adept at ensuring that clients, families, and communities are well informed and included in care planning and is an informed leader for improving care. The CNL also serves as an advocate for the profession and the interdisciplinary healthcare team.
Educator	Uses appropriate teaching principles and strategies as well as current information, materials, and technologies to teach clients, groups, and other healthcare professionals under their supervision.
Information manager	Able to use information systems and technology that put knowledge at the point of care to improve healthcare outcomes.
Systems analyst/risk anticipator	Able to participate in systems review to improve quality of client care delivery and at the individual level to critically evaluate and anticipate risks to client safety with the aim of preventing medical error.
Team manager	Able to properly delegate and manage the nursing team resources (human and fiscal) and serve as a leader and partner in the interdisciplinary healthcare team.
Member of a profession	Accountable for the ongoing acquisition of knowledge and skills to effect change in healthcare practice and outcomes and in the profession.
Lifelong learner	Recognizes the need for and actively pursues new knowledge and skills as one's role and needs of the healthcare system evolve.

Source: American Association of Colleges of Nursing. (2007). *White paper on the education and role of the clinical nurse leader* (p. 13). Washington, DC: Author.

patient outcome data to evaluate processes and procedures; communicates trends to administration and care team.
- **Systems analyst/risk anticipator:** Works with management when near misses/errors occur to determine cause and provide educational learning opportunities to the care team; analyzes outcomes and explores ways of improving processes; assesses daily patient risks for infection, pressure ulcers, pneumonia, and other nurse-driven indicators and takes steps to decrease risks; analyzes workflows to ensure smooth transition of care.
- **Team manager:** Coordinates and manages the interdisciplinary team; works with the entire team to confirm the overall plan of care focusing on individual patient needs; communicates all plans in a clear and detailed manner to the patient/family and team; collaborates with nurse manager to present patient/staff reports to administration.
- **Lifelong learner:** Maintains competence through continuing education in the area of heart failure and encourages staff to further their education by role modeling desire to learn; continuously searches for the most recent evidence and guidelines to manage heart failure patients.

The "What"

Basically, the "what" of your proposal is the development of the CNL position within the organization or unit. You have stated what the problem is and what you can do about it, and now you need to state that the CNL is the person/role that can address these issues and improve care and processes.

Go on to state that you are the best CNL to do this. You have gained the knowledge and skills from your CNL educational program to identify gaps in processes, initiate change, lead teams, and improve communication practices. You have the expertise in cardiac care to understand the physiologic condition, treatments, and patient characteristics of this population. The organization needs to hire you as the CNL to address the unit process concerns that are affecting care, retention of nurses, and ultimately the financial status of the unit.

If you get buy-in from the manager or other nurse leader, they can be your ally and guide you through your next steps. Remember, though, any organizational change requires time and work. You most likely will be required to develop a formal proposal. This proposal may include costs of the position, reporting structure, duties and responsibilities, organizational expectations, determining your effects on outcomes, and the return on investment for the organization.

If at first you do not get that positive response, do not give up! Reflect on your message and the manner in which you presented it to determine if you are really getting your point across and are highlighting factors most important to the administrators. Find a mentor—a leader who demonstrates qualities you admire. Meet with them and discuss how they are able to get their points across and create change. They may also be able to provide you with valuable insight into the culture of the organization and what the driving forces are at the moment that you can address in further discussions. Do not be afraid of failing—persistence will pay off in the end if you have the passion and drive to improve the healthcare systems.

Clinical Nurse Leader Vignette 1.1: Creating the Need for the Clinical Nurse Leader

I remember boldly discussing the CNL role with my boss and the CNO of my hospital prior to my graduation and certification. I wanted them to see my passion for the CNL role and how it could greatly affect patient care and staff satisfaction within my facility and especially within the ICU. They said, "Come and see us when you are all done with school; then we'll talk." I felt dejected and defeated, as though I had given a poor explanation of the role and how it could benefit my hospital, yet I had used all of the right buzzwords, like how I planned to "laterally integrate patient care," explained what an "advanced generalist" was, and discussed how I could be an "advocate for both patients and the healthcare team." What had I done wrong? Will I have to leave this facility before I can perform the role I had worked so hard to learn? How could I convince them CNLs were desperately needed in my facility?

Three months later, about a week before graduation and after I passed the CNL certification exam, I scheduled a meeting with those same two individuals. I reflected upon the positives of the earlier discussion and realized my reaction was the problem, not their comments. They could have easily said a swift "No!" when talking about CNL role implementation, but they did not. In fact, they left the door wide open for me to prove my worth as a CNL. And "worth" is the key word here. How much was it worth to them and the facility to have me perform this new role? I knew exactly what I had to do; show them what I had already done for the facility as a CNL student, what I could do for the ICU as a CNL employee, and how all of these activities equated to saving the facility money. There. I said it. Money. No more altruistic discussions about the touchy-feely side of nursing, but the hard, cold facts of 21st-century American healthcare wrapped within a portfolio showcasing the nine CNL roles. I started my new ICU CNL job a month later.

Ann Deerhake, DNP, RN, CNL, CCRN

DIFFERENTIATING YOUR ROLE FROM OTHER NURSING ROLES

Since the CNL is relatively new and not everyone is familiar with what you will bring to the table and how you are different from the other nursing roles within organizations, you may need to articulate the differences. You will need to describe how collaboratively each role works toward the betterment of the organization and care of the patients. Administrators do not always understand the fact that managers, educators, nurse practitioners, and clinical nurse specialists are not always at the point-of-care assisting nurses with their daily routines and overseeing care of the patient or how the point-of-care expert adds great value to the team. CNLs must be able to articulate these differences in order for administration to see that the CNL is a different position tending to different issues within the unit. Table 1.2 provides a brief overview of the various roles and their responsibilities.

Table 1.2

Differences Between Professional Nursing Roles and the Role of the Clinical Nurse Leader

Role	Clinical Nurse Leader
Manager	
■ Concentrates on budgets and overall business operations of the unit	■ Basic knowledge and understanding of microsystem finances
■ Hiring and disciplinary actions of staff	■ Manages resources
■ Not always at the point of care	■ Acts as resource and support for staff
■ Vertical management	■ Identifies staff educational needs

(continued)

Table 1.2

Differences Between Professional Nursing Roles and the Role of the Clinical Nurse Leader (*continued*)

Role	Clinical Nurse Leader
Clinical Nurse Specialist	
<ul><li>APRN</li><li>Works at the macro- or mesosystem</li><li>Involved in creating evidence and implements EBP through policy development</li><li>Involved in care delivery and planning for cohort of patients</li><li>Designs, implements, and evaluates programs of care to enhance patient outcomes across systems of care</li><li>Collaborates with interprofessional care teams throughout the meso/macrosystem</li></ul>	<ul><li>Advanced generalist</li><li>Works at the microsystem level</li><li>Responsible for utilization of evidence at the point of care</li><li>Performs comprehensive assessment of the patient/family/caregiver</li><li>Responsible for the ongoing assessment and modification of the plan of care and microsystem</li><li>Collaborates with the interprofessional team at the point of care</li></ul>
Certified Nurse Practitioner	
<ul><li>APRN</li><li>Trained in the process of diagnosing and treating medical conditions</li><li>Utilizes medical model of diagnosing and treating within their scope of practice</li><li>Autonomous independent practice under the licensure and professional credentials</li></ul>	<ul><li>Advanced generalist</li><li>Educated to complete advanced-level physical assessments beyond the level of the RN</li><li>Follows RN scope of practice</li><li>Authentic leader who does not function independently but under the direction of the facility and providers of care</li></ul>
Nurse Educator	
<ul><li>Generally works at the macrosystem level</li><li>Responsible for orientation/inservices</li><li>Educates in a more structured classroom setting</li><li>Provides education targeting competencies and overall learning needs of individual units or areas within an organization</li></ul>	<ul><li>Works at the microsystem level</li><li>Point-of-care educator to nurses/staff/interprofessional teams</li><li>Addresses individual employee educational needs</li><li>May collaborate with the nurse educator in identification of educational needs and educational programs</li></ul>

EBP, evidence-based practice.

ELEVATOR SPEECH

You may have been introduced to the elevator speech and had an assignment to create one during your schooling. If you did, be sure to pull it out of your files and practice it. If you have not developed one, do it now. It will be extremely important to be able to quickly articulate who you are and what you do for patients, staff, and the interprofessional team. If you are just beginning on your unit as a CNL, the care team may be wondering what your role actually is and how you fit into the team. It will also be important if you are in a meeting with administrators to tell them exactly what you do in just a minute or two. An example of an elevator speech may be, "Hi, I'm Susie the CNL on 11 East. I am an advanced generalist registered nurse at the point of care, coordinating patients and families with all healthcare team members and their associated resources, in an effort to create a patent-centered, transdisciplinary team. These coordination activities increase patient satisfaction and practitioner collaboration, leading to positive patient outcomes. Additionally, they decrease facility-acquired infections, falls, pressure ulcers, and many other negative outcomes, thereby decreasing healthcare costs and once again, boosting patient and provider satisfaction as a whole." Be sure to practice your speech a few times so you can state it quickly, articulating the high points of what you do.

Creating a Portfolio

Nurses may be familiar with portfolios which were a requirement during their educational programs, as many colleges of nursing require them as a means of documenting completed educational competencies and skills. Portfolios, however, are not widely used by professional nurses. As you move forward in your career as a nursing leader, it is important for you to document your professional accomplishments in order to demonstrate experience and skill to administrators and peers. It is also important for you to keep track of your activities for relicensure and recertification purposes.

A portfolio should highlight what you have done in the past. For example, what leadership activities have you been involved with? What committees have you worked on and chaired? What continuing education have you attended or even developed and presented? Have you written any published works? Have you presented at conferences? What quality improvement activities have you worked on? Have you precepted or mentored new nurses or students? All of these accomplishments demonstrate activities that go above and beyond your normal daily activities and demonstrate as well professional

Table 1.3

Clinical Nurse Leader (CNL) Resources

CNL Resources

AACN General CNL Site	https://www.aacnnursing.org/CNL
AACN Education and Practice Site	https://www.aacnnursing.org/CNL/Education-Practice-Resources
AACN Competencies and Curricular Expectations for the Clinical Nurse Leader (includes the White Paper)	https://www.aacnnursing.org/Portals/42/AcademicNursing/CurriculumGuidelines/CNL-Competencies-October-2013.pdf
AACN Career Services Site	https://www.aacnnursing.org/CNL-Certification/CNL-Career-Services
CNL Career Resource Guide	https://www.aacnnursing.org/Portals/42/CNL/CNL-Resource-Guide.pdf
AACN/CNC The Clinical Nurse Leader "Why Hire a CNL" Brochure	https://www.aacnnursing.org/Portals/42/CNL/Evolving-Role-of-CNL.pdf
AACN Clinical Nurse Leader Tool Kit	https://www.aacnnursing.org/Education-Resources/Tool-Kits/Clinical-Nurse-Leader-Tool-Kit
Clinical Nurse Leader Association	https://cnlassociation.org/
CNC "Discover the Valuable Impact of the Certified CNL"	http://discovercnls.org/where-cnls-practice/

AACN, American Association of Colleges of Nursing; CNC, Commission on Nurse Certification.

growth and accountability. You may also want to maintain a listing of the outcomes you have contributed to in patient safety and outcomes that have contributed positively to the organization. Demonstrating your worth to the organization is instrumental for CNLs in sustaining their positions. Organizations evaluate positions and processes often when looking at their overall financial status. CNLs must demonstrate their value by keeping track of what they do and their overall benefit to the organization.

Think about how you currently keep track of what you do and how you can organize to maintain better records. It can be as easy as purchasing a three-ring binder with paper protectors. Place your continuing education certificates in the binder along with any thank you notes or recognition certificates. When working on projects, keep outlines of what the project is, the steps you have taken throughout the project, your contributions to the project, and especially the outcomes. These documents will be invaluable to you as you proceed in your career, demonstrating growth and potential to future employers and administrators.

RESOURCES

As you progress in your career as a CNL, keep in mind that there are resources to help you along the way. It is not always easy being a pioneer, but remember, you are a much needed discipline to patients and organizations. Your expertise, skills, and knowledge will improve practice, processes, and outcomes. The AACN (2018a) website has a section on career services, which will provide you with documents such as a resource guide and CNL talking points to help in compiling information to deliver the best speech ever. (See Table 1.3 for a complete listing.) The Clinical Nurse Leader Association is a professional organization for CNLs and CNL students that also offers resources and insight into what is happening in the CNL community. Stay connected with your classmates and peers who have gone on to positions in other organizations and attend conferences to get to know CNLs throughout the country. Be sure to network with as many CNLs as possible to help you achieve your dreams of changing healthcare for the better.

References

American Association of Colleges of Nursing. (2007). *White paper on the education and role of the clinical nurse leader.* Washington, DC: Author.

American Association of Colleges of Nursing. (2018a). *CNL career services.* Retrieved from https://www.aacnnursing.org/CNL-Certification/CNL-Career-Services

American Association of Colleges of Nursing. (2018b). *CNL certification.* Retrieved from https://www.aacnnursing.org/CNL-Certification

Bender, M. (2014). The current evidence base for the clinical nurse leader: A narrative review of the literature. *Journal of Professional Nursing, 30*(2), 110–123. doi:10.1016/j.profnurs.2013.08.006

Case-Wirth, J. (2018, February). *Hardwiring the CNL role into complex healthcare environments.* Paper presented at the American Association of Colleges of Nursing, 2018 CNL. Summit, Garden Grove, CA.

Commission on Nurse Certification. (2017). *A national snapshot of where CNLs practice.* Retrieved from http://discovercnls.org/where-cnls-practice/

Hix, C., McKeon, L., & Walters, S. (2009). Clinical nurse leader impact on clinical microsystems outcomes. *The Journal of Nursing Administration, 39*(2), 71–76. doi:10.1097/NNA.0b013e318195a612

Institute of Medicine. (1999). *To err is human: Building a safer health system.* Washington, DC: The National Academies Press.

Institute of Medicine. (2000). *Crossing the quality chasm. A new health system for the 21st century.* Washington, DC: The National Academies Press.

Lahmiri, S. (2016). Economic decision-making, emotion, and prefrontal cortex. In B. Christiansen & E. Lechman (Eds.), *Neuroeconomics and the decision making process* (pp. 122–131). Retrieved from https://ebookcentral-proquest-com.proxy.lib.ohio-state.edu

Makary, M., & Daniel, M. (2016). Medical error—the third leading cause of death in the U.S. *BMJ, 353*, 1–5. doi:10.1136/bmj.i2139

Moore, P. (2013). The academic story: Introducing the clinical nurse leader role in a multifacility health care system. *Journal of Professional Nursing, 29*(5), 264–269. doi:10.1016/j.profnurs.2012.10.007

Ott, K., Haddock, K. S., Fox, S. E., Shinn, J. K., Walters, S. E., Hardin, J. W., … Harris, J. L. (2009). The clinical nurse leader: Impact on practice outcomes in the Veterans Health Administration. *Nursing Economics, 27*(6), 363–383.

Ousdal, O., Specht, K., Server, A., Andreassen, O. A., Dolan, R. J., & Jensen, J. (2014). The human amygdala encodes value and space during decision making. *NeuroImage, 101*, 712–719. doi:10.1016/j.neuroimage.2014.07.005

Rankin, V., Ralyea, T., & Sotomayor, G. (2017). Clinical nurse leaders forging the path of population health. *Journal of Professional Nursing, 34*, 269–272. doi:10.1016/j.profnurs.2017.10.008

Sinek, S. (2009). *Start with why*. London, UK: Penguin Books.

Sinek, S. (2014). *How great leaders inspire action* [Video file]. Retrieved from https://www.ted.com/talks/simon_sinek_how_great_leaders_inspire_action?utm_campaign=tedspread&utm_medium=referral&utm_source=tedcomshare

Sotomayor, G., & Rankin, V. (2017). Clinical nurse leaders: Fulfilling the promise of the role. *MEDSURG Nursing, 26*(1), 21–32.

Sternberg, S. (2016, May 3). Medical errors are third leading cause of death in the U.S. *U.S. News & World Report*. Retrieved from https://www.usnews.com/news/articles/2016-05-03/medical-errors-are-third-leading-cause-of-death-in-the-us

U.S. Department of Veterans Affairs. (n.d.). *Office of Nursing Services: Clinical Nurse Leader*. Retrieved from https://www.va.gov/NURSING/practice/cnl.asp

2

Integration Into Clinical Nurse Leader Practice: Preparing to Lead

Ann Deerhake

"Journal writing gives us insights into who we are, who we were, and who we can become."

~Sandra Marinella

INTRODUCTION

You have advocated for the clinical nurse leader (CNL) role within your facility and obtained the position of your dreams. It is finally time to move into CNL practice and launch your new role. Where do you begin? Perhaps the most important starting point is reflecting upon what you have done to achieve this career milestone. Remind yourself of the hard work and dedication it took to achieve this goal, such as studying constantly, missing family time, losing sleep, and anything else that comes to mind. Now, write all of these sacrifices down as your first entry in a "My CNL Journey" journal, using whatever form of readily available reflection that works best for you, whether electronic file, blog, mobile app, or pen and paper. This journal will become a source of comfort as well as a usable tool to develop and maintain your role. This chapter provides a guide for implementation and maintenance of CNL practice, including tools for microsystem assessment and daily practice.

After reading this chapter, you will be able to:

1. Identify strategies for transitioning into the CNL role
2. Individualize the CNL role to a variety of healthcare settings
3. Manage the CNL role in your microsystem
4. Articulate the importance of professional, microsystem, and organizational goal alignment
5. Synthesize strategies to track infusion of roles into daily practice

TRANSITIONING INTO THE CNL ROLE

Role Transition for the New Nurse

The direct-entry CNL, the nurse who has entered nursing as a CNL without previous nursing experience, has the advantage of bringing fewer preconceived ideas of nursing to the role, all the while applying real-life common sense and newly gained knowledge of healthcare systems to the application of the role. Nurses of all preparation and skill levels share the common bond of wanting to provide compassionate, competent care for patients and, at the same time, constantly assess the ability of others to do so as well. A new nurse in a new role of CNL may appear threatening to those who have more clinical nursing experience, especially to nurses who have been working in the same microsystem for a long time. Some staff may try to test the CNL's clinical or administrative knowledge by questioning the CNL's rationale for practice, whereas others will quietly, but critically, observe.

Assessing the nursing structure of your new setting is instrumental in determining how to succeed within the particular microsystem culture. Questions to explore include the following: Who are the managerial leaders? Who are the point-of-care (POC) leaders? Is nurse-to-nurse communication healthy? What barriers exist for new nurses? After reflecting upon the answers to these questions, consider how you will begin to build rapport with the staff. Advocating for a healthy work environment (HWE) begins by using "skilled communication, true collaboration, effective decision making, appropriate staffing, meaningful recognition and authentic leadership" (American Association of Critical-Care Nurses, 2016, para. 10). Take the time to listen critically and communicate clearly; you will never get the chance to make a first impression again. Be strong in your conviction regarding what you know, but be collaborative and willing to learn when dealing with things you do not know. Knowing when to be leader and when to be a follower is an important distinction.

Essential Facts

Being a good follower is as important as being a good leader. Through intentional following, you become aware of what distresses or inspires others.

Building Team Relationships

Building relationships with other staff members is extremely important in being an active member of the team. Grossman and Valiga (2017) remark that team leaders hone relationships by bonding teams together, and as a CNL who wishes to be a genuine leader, your goal is to be that glue. The relationships you create will enhance your ability to generate change to improve practice and outcomes. You will need to have allies in your quest for improvements, and those allies come through the relationships you create. You most likely have determined who the natural unit leaders are, so take time to get to know them better and build that trusting relationship. Building trust requires time and requires you to earn the trust of others. Be truthful and make sure you can keep any promises you make. Be willing to assist when times are rough, and maintain a positive demeanor without being harsh or belittling when approaching others. Acknowledge others for their accomplishments, and be encouraging to those who are unsure of their abilities.

Following staff and learning the intricacies of the unit permit you to gain an understanding of issues that arise which may impede staff from performing essential tasks. Following also allows staff to see that you are really interested in helping them and not just attempting to change their routines. Ask questions of staff regarding how they perceive their work and what they feel are impediments to their care processes. Asking questions allows them to see that you are really interested in their input. Assisting staff in care by helping with dressing changes, line care, and any other skills permits them to see that you are not administration handing down edicts; you are there to support them and enhance care.

Listening to the staff is also an important skill. Being an active listener is when you are not just hearing the words of another, but you are actually processing the message sent. This may take practice in avoiding outside distractions and inner thoughts from clouding the message. Rephrasing their message is a good method of ensuring you have understood their concerns accurately. Listen attentively to their concerns, and ask them for their opinions or solutions. As stated previously, asking them for their ideas for solutions permits them to feel you are interested in their points of view and may help with the relationship-building process.

Role Transition for the Experienced Nurse

The experienced nurse starting as a novice CNL in an unfamiliar setting may encounter many of the same issues as a direct-entry CNL. Although you may possess a wealth of clinical experience and knowledge, implementing and performing the CNL role is a brand-new career path for you. Assessing the microsystem nursing structure and working to build rapport with staff is critical; do not think you can skip this step because you have been a nurse for a long time. Consider your past behavior when new nurses came to work alongside you: How did you react to a new person on the unit, and what coworker criteria did you need them to meet to fully embrace them as a team member? Now, translate that into your current situation with you being the new nurse entering the unit in a different, perhaps not fully understood, role. Initiate clear communication with your elevator speech, and be prepared to educate others on your specific role within the microsystem, starting with how your role will affect and enhance their practice.

Additionally, the experienced nurse starting as a new CNL within a familiar microsystem may need to take a different approach than the direct-entry CNL. Unlike those who are unfamiliar with the setting, the nursing structure is known, and staff rapport is in place, albeit in the context of a non-CNL role. The difficult issue here is establishing yourself as a CNL, and it will require educating others on how this change will affect their relationship with you, as well as their professional role and work environment. Once again, a well-developed elevator speech is critical, but no more important than further dialogue regarding your specific new role within this particular microsystem. It can be difficult for nursing staff to understand why you, the experienced nurse who knows this setting well, do not take a patient assignment when they need help. Therefore, establishing your role by being mindful and showing others exactly what you do and how it affects their practice is crucial. This understanding on the part of the staff takes time to develop. One way to facilitate this process is by offering to help and collaborate at the bedside, which not only keeps clinical skills intact but allows the bedside nurse to see mutual goal alignment. Be the support person by contacting medical providers, performing skills, or defusing conflicts, which will ultimately enhance CNL role acceptance.

UNDERSTANDING THE CNL ROLE WITHIN SPECIFIC HEALTHCARE SETTINGS

Wherever healthcare consumers seek healthcare, a CNL is needed. Given that the CNL discipline includes the roles of clinician, educator, and patient advocate, it makes sense that the CNL role should be implemented throughout healthcare settings. All nine CNL role components will be utilized differently and in varying percentages, based on the current goals and needs of the facility and the experience and skill level of the CNL. The most important consideration here is staying true to the CNL role; spending all of your time performing only one or two components of the role does not make a CNL! Learning to build your role by taking on activities that fulfill all components of the role will brand you as well versed and indispensable.

Acute Care

The American Association of Colleges of Nursing's (AACN; 2013) CNL white paper discusses the need for CNLs "across the continuum of care within any healthcare setting in today's changing healthcare environment" (p. 4). Much of the published literature, however, speaks to the role of CNLs within various hospital microsystems, including oncology, intensive care, and pediatric settings. Hospitalized patients are perhaps the most complex people receiving care, requiring assistance with clinical care, educational needs, risk reduction, and information management throughout their hospital stay and after discharge. Additionally, the constantly changing acute care environment requires that bedside staff be educated frequently, supported by team resources and empowered as members of the nursing profession. To perform all of these skills successfully, the CNL must be an organized and observant leader.

The primary role of a CNL in acute care is to clinically optimize the function of a microsystem as evidenced by moving patients efficiently and seamlessly through different levels of care. As the unit CNL, your goal should be to reduce communication silos by facilitating lateral integration among the entire patient-led healthcare team, coordinating care, thereby improving patient outcomes (L'Ecuyer, Shatto, Hoffmann, & Crecelius, 2016). First, the CNL assesses the microsystem (see the section "Microsystem Needs"), finding the broken process patterns. Talking with nursing staff and unit management is an important part of this assessment, as it is amazing what you can discover in simple, informal conversations. Next, although gaps in care will likely be many, the CNL must choose the top three issues and work to alleviate them. Try to pick issues that correspond with three different CNL roles, such as the need for (a) clinical assistance to help find a resolution for a problematic procedure; (b) risk reduction of such issues as patient pressure ulcers, falls, or hospital-acquired infection; and (c) education development for your microsystem's most frequently prescribed medications. Countless other issues will arise, and your services will be requested; however, this work must be your priority, along with your daily routine of assisting the healthcare team and patients with POC needs. Within your journal, keep a list of these requests, and when you repair one issue, start on the next. You will soon learn how much you can handle and how much more you can take on.

Emergency/Ambulatory Care

Providing quick yet complete care is the goal of EDs around the country. Ambulatory care and outpatient settings aspire to deliver procedural care in an individualized, proficient manner. In these settings, the primary role of CNLs is to clinically optimize a microsystem as evidenced by moving patients efficiently and seamlessly through procedures, treatments, and discharges. They also collaborate with bedside nurses and physicians to coordinate care with the receiving unit if a patient requires inpatient admission, as well as locate needed community resources for those being discharged. CNLs can also provide knowledgeable support and advocacy to families and friends of patients, especially those in crisis.

Rankin, Ralyea, and Sotomayor (2018) discuss innovative CNL roles, including CNLs in different ED settings working on patient flow issues by collaboratively creating a process to balance the patient population of tertiary and community EDs, as well as inpatient and outpatient high-risk obstetric CNLs working together to coordinate care for this high-acuity population throughout pregnancy and postpartum. Identifying process gaps and system issues within your proposed ambulatory practice setting will provide support for the need to employ a CNL to remedy these problems, improving patient care and saving money simultaneously. Once again, performing a microsystem assessment and talking with staff is key in determining the needs of the unit and thereby your role.

Essential Facts

The Dartmouth Institute Microsystem Academy provides free inpatient and outpatient microsystem assessment tools at http://clinicalmicrosystem.org/knowledge-center/workbooks.

Primary Care

Although most of the published CNL literature highlights CNLs within acute care, it is reasonable to consider their likely positive impact on primary care. This setting can be influenced by the systems knowledge, lateral integration, health promotion, and disease prevention skills a CNL possesses to improve health outcomes. According to the American Academy of Family Physicians (AAFP; 2018), primary care practices are the first place many consumers seek healthcare, giving them the unique opportunity to offer a multitude of services that assist patients in developing a comprehensive plan of care. In recent years, patient-centered medical homes (PCMHs) have been established via primary care practices and settings, with the goal of providing patients with care that is "comprehensive, patient-centered, coordinated, accessible and safe" (Agency for Healthcare Research and Quality [AHRQ], 2018). While current primary care structures may not frequently utilize the CNL role to direct the PCMH, you can present a business case for the role by showcasing the need for the CNL skill set to effectively coordinate these programs. PCMHs, done correctly, are lofty initiatives requiring the services of a generalist professional who can integrate and assess the work of the healthcare team, expose gaps in treatment and provide solutions, as well as work closely with patients to determine needs.

Essential Facts

A PCMH is not just a place where a patient receives care but a framework that practitioners can use to make sure they are meeting all of the patient's care needs (AHRQ, 2018).

Community Health

According to the National Academies of Medicine (2013) (formerly the Institute of Medicine [IOM]), the simplest definition of population health may be "community well-being"; however, they also discuss that it may be more accurate to say population health is about working toward improving outcomes for groups of people by identifying and assessing their specific determinants of health. Any way you define it, improving health from a population perspective is one of the biggest topics in healthcare currently and the wave of the future, especially for the aging U.S. population. From a CNL standpoint, education regarding the roles of patient advocate and outcome manager prepares the CNL to work at the population level.

By applying the CNL's expert systems knowledge, you can transform community health settings into high-performing microsystems, creating a public healthcare mesosystem of healthcare professionals who can share information and evidence-based practice (EBP) initiatives, as well as provide patients with community POC resources. Additionally, you can also advocate for implementation of the CNL role within the patient's home environment. Stocker-Schneider (2014) discusses that CNLs are a great fit in home care, and their integration of care, team, and process management skills enables them to lead care effectively within the home.

Essential Facts

Within the next 20 years, more people in the United States will be older than age 65, surpassing the number of children less than 18 years of age (U.S. Census Bureau, 2018).

MANAGING THE ROLE

Starting a new role within a busy healthcare setting can be a daunting task, even more so if the role is also new to the facility. The goal is to build a routine that is reasonable for you to perform, yet effective for your microsystem. You can begin by breaking down CNL responsibilities into a manageable format, such as listing your professional needs, microsystem needs, and organizational needs. Once again, your journal can come in handy here!

Your Needs

One of the most important components of developing your CNL role to satisfy your professional needs is the concept of self-management. This includes determining your current CNL strengths and weaknesses, as well as designing a professional work action plan to maintain and build your skills. Using templates for each of these tasks, such as those available at https://www.smartsheet.com/14-free-swot-analysis-templates and https://www.smartsheet.com/develop-plan-action-free-templates (Eby, 2016a, 2016b), can help you gain insight about yourself both personally and professionally. To ensure that you gain experience in all of the CNL roles, make sure you analyze your project role based on not only the needs of the unit but also your personal growth. Also, planning networking activities, such as attending conferences or working on committees with other CNL professionals and facility nurses is a must. Time spent collaboratively learning with others creates professional bonds you can use to reach out for ideas, support, and advice.

While some CNL roles may be paid on an hourly basis, most are paid a salary. Many nurses are subjecting themselves to their first salaried position when starting a CNL job, including the inflexibility of the 5-day work week and yet the flexibility of setting your own hours each day. Determining your own work schedule can be difficult when experience has taught you only the rigidity of others deciding your work hours for you. Understanding your responsibility to yourself both personally and professionally is important. As you complete your microsystem assessment, you will begin to understand its flow, helping you to plan your routine, including a daily time frame for your work. While flexibility is nice, set hours are important so others know when you are available to them and, more importantly, when you are not. This process takes planning, continuous reassessment, and modification, similar to a PDSA (plan-do-study-act) cycle.

Essential Facts

You can create your own personal weekly PDSA cycle!
Plan: Write down your schedule for the week. Use your journal or an online calendar.
Do: Follow your schedule!
Study: Each day, answer the question "How did my schedule work for me today?" Don't feel bad if you didn't accomplish everything you wanted; be realistic, not discouraged!
Act: Make changes (including delegation!) as needed and try it again!

Setting goals is a critical step in determining your professional needs. Managing yourself and your time will be easier to do if you set short-term and long-term goals. Short-term goals can include interacting with and building relationships with microsystem staff, educating others on the role of the CNL, and showcasing how your function is different from the roles of bedside nurse and nurse manager. Long-term goals could include establishing yourself as a process expert, evidence-based practice (EBP) implementer, healthcare team collaborator, and money saver. One way to do this is to complete, publish, and present a microsystem quality improvement project, highlighting the results by calculating the return on investment (ROI).

Microsystem Needs

Microsystem observation is the initial step in determining microsystem needs. Those needs will comprise the foundation of the CNL role within this setting. For example, if staff knowledge deficits are noted, procuring and/or developing education will be a part of the CNL role. If multiple faulty processes are observed, then risk assessments and system analysis will be a large part of the CNL role. If dissemination of information to patients and staff is poor, then managing information effectively will become a part of the CNL role. It is unrealistic to think that all CNL roles will be performed evenly all of the time; this is not true in any microsystem. The flexibility and advanced generalist nature of the CNL role is its benefit. Building the CNL role to fit your specific microsystem will allow you to become an expert within this particular setting.

After a few days of observation, complete a microsystem assessment to organize needs in your mind, as well as communicate those needs to others. Completing a 5P assessment will categorize the microsystem and expose problems, allowing you to focus on many small areas of needed improvement as well as short- and long-term goal setting. The 5P assessment (see Figure 2.1) includes analyzing your microsystem's:

- Purpose: Why does this microsystem exist?
- Patients: Who does the microsystem serve?
- Professionals: What members of the healthcare team work here, and why?
- Processes: What are the most frequent processes used here?
- Patterns: Have patterns emerged concerning safety, patient/staff satisfaction, or costs?

Based on the results of this assessment, teams will be formed, responsibilities determined, rules established, and goals set. This book provides more in-depth discussion of the microsystem assessment.

The 6S Assessment is another way to analyze your microsystem (Figure 2.2). This type of assessment looks at reducing waste and improving productivity. Provided by the Environmental Protection Agency (EPA) (2006, p. 5), the concepts and questions considered here are more geared toward the environment of care and include the following:

- Sort: What items are needed/not needed? Rid the area of what you do not need.
- Set in order: What is left organized and in place?
- Shine: Have items that are left been inspected and deemed clean?

- Standardize: Are there standard processes in place to maintain cleanliness and safety?
- Sustain: Do employees follow established rules to sustain the organized environment?
- Safety: Is the environment safe for all?

This assessment exposes and categorizes safety, personnel, and environmental issues, yielding a definitive plan that can be used to sustain a safe and productive environment of care.

Short-term goals for microsystem improvement can include daily rounding at the POC, attending unit-based meetings, discussing current quality improvement with nurse managers, interacting with staff regarding process gaps, and establishing yourself as the contact person for patient questions or educational needs. Achieving these goals is just the beginning of building a high-performing microsystem, as they are activities that lead to larger initiatives. Long-term goals generally include these larger initiatives, such as reducing hospital-acquired infection, facilitating patient throughput, and increasing staff retention.

Organizational Needs

The final step in managing your new CNL role is *aligning goals* with your organization as a whole. Answer the questions "What is the true mission of my organization?" and "What are the hot topics that concern both the administration of my facility and my microsystem?" Identifying these issues and then aligning goals among you as the CNL, your specific microsystem, and your facility's administration are critical to the current success and longevity of the CNL role. To do this, the CNL must be observational in demeanor, yet intentional when discussing issues with administrators, frequently introducing the three prongs of EBP into the conversation, including the importance of utilizing the best literature, clinical expertise, and patient preferences.

INFUSION OF ROLES INTO DAILY PRACTICE

With goals in hand, it is time to start the implementation of the CNL role on a daily basis, posing the question "Where do I start?" Taking the leap into actual CNL practice is difficult; therefore, having the tools you have created, such as an elevator speech, SWOT (strengths, weaknesses, opportunities, and threats) analysis, microsystem assessment, and planned activity schedule readily accessible,

Microsystem Name

Purpose/AIM

Patients

People with healthcare needs

People with healthcare needs met

Functional & Risks ⊕ Expectations
Biological ⊕ Costs

Functional & Risks ⊕ Satisfaction
Biological ⊕ Costs

- (P) Prevention
- (A) Acute
- (C) Chronic
- (PP) Palliative
- (E) Educate

P A C PP E — Very High Risk
P A C PP E — Chronic
P A E — Healthy
Palliative

Processes

Professionals

STAFF MEMBERS:

_____ _____
_____ _____
_____ _____
_____ _____
_____ _____
_____ _____

Skill Mix: MDs __ RNs __ NP/PAs __ MA __ LPN __ SECs __

Performance Patterns

Measuring Team Performance & Patient Outcomes and Costs

Measure	Current	Target	Measure	Current	Target
Panel Size Adj.			External Referral Adj. PMPM-Team		
Direct Pt. Care Hours: MD/Assoc.			Patient Satisfaction		
% Panel Seeing Own PCP:			Access Satisfaction		
Total PMPM Adj. PMPM-Team			Staff Satisfaction		

Figure 2.1 The 5P Wall Model: Analyzing the purpose, patients, professionals, processes, and patterns of the microsystem.

Note: Microsystem Approach 6/17/1998. Revised: March 2004.

Source: © Eugene C. Nelson, DSc, MPH, and Paul B. Batalden, MD, Dartmouth-Hitchcock Clinic, June 1998. The Dartmouth Institute Microsystem Academy. (2004). *5 Ps Wall Model.* Retrieved from http://clinicalmicrosystem.org/knowledge-center/worksheets.

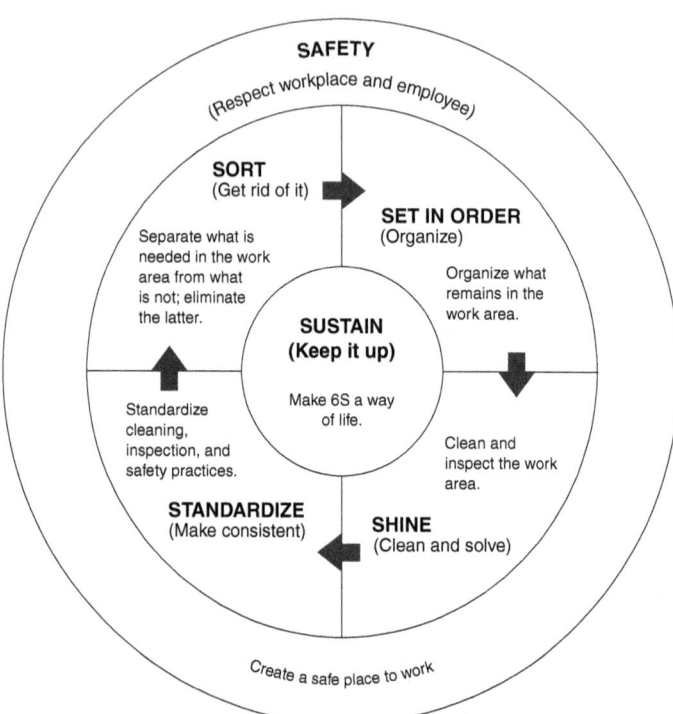

Figure 2.2 The 6S assessment: analyzing microsystems to reduce waste and improve productivity.

Source: Environmental Protection Agency. (2006). *Lean and environmental training modules*. Retrieved from https://www.epa.gov/sites/production/files/2015-06/documents/module_5_6s.pdf

is important. Sharing these metrics and assessment tools with others highlights your commitment to professional practice, as well as your skill as a CNL; applying them will create a needs-based microsystem plan for improvement.

Developing a Needs-Based Plan

The first step in developing a needs-based plan is goal prioritization. It is not likely that only one problem has resulted from your microsystem assessment, so determining which issues are priorities is important. Generally, those process problems that directly impact patient care as well as create reimbursement issues are the first to be rectified, such as high rates of pressure ulcers, hospital-acquired infections, falls, and low rates of patient satisfaction. All members of the healthcare team will benefit from improving these issues, especially patients. The next sets of goals to be addressed are facility-wide initiatives, such as nurse education and retention and global patient safety. Finally, microsystem-specific goals can be evaluated, such as alarm fatigue reduction and increased effectiveness of bedside patient education.

When working toward collaborative goal alignment among the organization, microsystem, and CNL practitioner, developing a CNL role component–based intervention plan can be a sensible strategy. Many organizations wish to place CNLs in jobs that only utilize a small portion of their skill set; therefore, defining and individualizing each of the nine CNL role components within the microsystem, along with how they can be utilized to reach the established goals, will set up a framework to guide CNL practice. This intervention plan can also be a tool you can use to educate those who are unfamiliar with the components of the CNL role. Tracking which of the CNL role components you commonly perform gives you a visual representation of how well-rounded your role truly is, and allows for addition or delegation of interventions, based on the frequency of components used. Table 2.1 illustrates a simple role component–based intervention plan.

Table 2.1

Role Component–Based Intervention Plan for Clinical Nurse Leader Practice

Role Component	Example Intervention	Goal
Clinician	Encourage nursing staff daily to monitor devices and maintain every 2-hr turns	Reduce pressure ulcers in ICU
Outcomes manager	Meet with lab and ICU staff monthly to determine barriers to blood culture turnaround times	Decrease the delay in blood culture result process in ICU
Client advocate	Assess patients twice weekly for pressure ulcers and assist with turns	Reduce pressure ulcers in ICU
Educator	Provide information and one-to-one counseling regarding clinical ladder requirements weekly	Empower ICU staff to apply for clinical ladder program

(continued)

Table 2.1

Role Component–Based Intervention Plan for Clinical Nurse Leader Practice (*continued*)

Role Component	Example Intervention	Goal
Information manager	Disseminate information regarding accurate labeling of blood cultures within the weekly e-update	Decrease the delay in blood culture result process in ICU
Systems analyst Risk anticipator	Collaborate with nursing staff to assess patients for pressure ulcer risk on admission and daily	Reduce pressure ulcers in ICU
Team manager	Organize and meet monthly with a transdisciplinary team to examine pressure ulcer issues	Reduce pressure ulcers in ICU
Member of a profession	Encourage nurses to reflect on their practice and how it relates to clinical ladder initiatives	Empower ICU staff to apply for clinical ladder program
Lifelong learner	Role-model application of EBP to practice via biweekly journal club offerings	Empower ICU staff to apply for clinical ladder program

EBP, evidence-based practice.

Clinical Nurse Leader Vignette 2.1: A Day in the Life of a CNL Within a Cardiovascular Surgery Microsystem

Although CNL roles look quite different from setting to setting, following is a real-life example of the CNL role in action. This CNL's role focuses on care coordination, risk assessment, quality improvement, transitions/communication of care, patient/staff satisfaction, and patient education needs.

Time	Activity	Focus
6:00 a.m.	*Peripheral vascular surgeons' (PVS) rounds*	- Pain, labs, BM regimen, OOB, IS, progression and tentative discharge date, discharge needs, engage bedside RNs in rounds

Time	Activity	Focus
	Room safety/quality check	- IV tubings labeled, curos caps in place, dressings, and IV dressings dated
7:00 a.m.	Safety huddle and charge RN report	- Relay PVS updates to charge RN
7:30 a.m.	Chart review Staff rounds Project work	- Appropriate care plans selected, patient portal tablets given, teletracking and update, review acuity, MEWS scores and readmission risk scores - Address/follow-up staff concerns, relay PVS updates, check empty rooms for safety and key supplies, remove extra supplies, and check for room repairs - Work on unit projects for education/workflow
9:30 a.m.	Interdisciplinary rounds with PT/OT, SW, CM, PVS intern/NP and patients	- Review reason for admission, progression and discharge planning, anticoagulation, lines, and drains - Review needs, f/u appointments, SNF/LTACH placement, home health, medical equipment - Relay information to bedside nurse
10:15 a.m.	Readiness reviews Nurse leader rounds Bedside nurse assist	- Review teletracking, LOS, and discharges for readiness - Complete rounds with unit hospital leadership - Second assist with post-op patients, ERTs, codes
12:00 p.m.	Lunch	- Or CNL meeting or grand rounds
12:30–1:00 p.m.	Follow-up Project work	- Update staff with labs, orders, PVS requests - Discharge needs, timeliness - Safety and supply needs check - Work on unit projects for education/workflow
2:30 p.m.	Leave for the day	

References

Agency for Healthcare Research and Quality. (2018). *Defining the PCMH*. Retrieved from https://pcmh.ahrq.gov/page/defining-pcmh

American Academy of Family Physicians. (2018). *Primary care*. Retrieved from https://www.aafp.org/about/policies/all/primary-care.html

American Association of Colleges of Nursing. (2013). *Competencies and curricular expectations for the clinical nurse leader in education and practice*. Retrieved from https://www.aacnnursing.org/Portals/42/News/White-Papers/CNL-Competencies-October-2013.pdf

American Association of Critical-Care Nurses. (2016). *AACN standards for establishing and sustaining healthy work environments: Executive summary*. Retrieved from https://www.aacn.org/~/media/aacn-website/nursing-excellence/healthy-work-environment/execsum.pdf?la=en

The Dartmouth Institute Microsystem Academy. (2004). *5 Ps Wall Model*. Retrieved from http://clinicalmicrosystem.org/knowledge-center/worksheets

Eby, K. (2016a). *Develop a plan of action with free templates*. Retrieved from https://www.smartsheet.com/develop-plan-action-free-templates

Eby, K. (2016b). *14 Free SWOT analysis templates*. Retrieved from https://www.smartsheet.com/14-free-swot-analysis-templates

Environmental Protection Agency. (2006). *Lean and environmental training modules*. Retrieved from https://www.epa.gov/sites/production/files/2015-06/documents/module_5_6s.pdf

Grossman, S., & Valiga, T. (2017). *The new leadership challenge creating the future of nursing*. Philadelphia, PA: F. A. Davis Company.

L'Ecuyer, K., Shatto, B., Hoffmann, R., & Crecelius, M. (2016). The certified clinical nurse leader in critical care. *Dimensions of Critical Care Nursing: DCCN*, 35(5), 248–254. doi:10.1097/DCC.0000000000000202

National Academies of Medicine. (2013). *Working definition of population health*. Retrieved from https://www.nationalacademies.org/documents/link/web?IdcService=GET_FILE&dLinkID=LD2305695AFDBC7E10E384EC8DB77A9CC3943CC47EC1&item=fFileGUID%3aD364E62969252C3EB23005257E505B5E707C6FE239E4&scsOriginalFileName=Pop%20Health%20RT%20Population%20Health%20Working%20Definition.pdf

Rankin, V., Ralyea, T., & Sotomayor, G. (2018). Clinical Nurse Leaders forging the path of population health. *Journal of Professional Nursing*, 34(4), 269–272. doi:10.1016/j.profnurs.2017.10.008

Stocker-Schneider, J. (2014). Clinical nurse leader. *Home Healthcare Nurse*, 32(9), 563–564. doi:10.1097/NHH.0000000000000146

U.S. Census Bureau. (2018). *Older people projected to outnumber children for first time in U.S. history*. Retrieved from https://www.census.gov/newsroom/press-releases/2018/cb18-41-population-projections.html

3

Leadership Within a Complex Environment

Janice Wilcox

"Invention, it must be humbly admitted, does not consist in creating out of void but out of chaos."

~Mary Shelley

INTRODUCTION

Today's healthcare systems are complex with many interacting parts that impact how nurses and interdisciplinary teams care for patients as well as how leaders lead. Leading within this complexity requires an understanding of the theoretical underpinnings of chaos, complexity, and systems thinking to determine how these concepts affect work, outcomes, and leadership. Exploring changes that have occurred over the years provides insight of the evolution of healthcare and of the complexity that has ensued. It is beneficial for the clinical nurse leader (CNL) to be knowledgeable of all of the factors that affect how one leads within microsystems today.

After reading this chapter, you will be able to:

1. Describe changes in today's healthcare system
2. Apply characteristics of chaos and complexity to healthcare organizations
3. Determine differences in traditional and complexity leadership styles
4. Incorporate leadership styles within a complex system

Leadership is a "multi-faceted process of identifying a goal, motivating other people to act, and providing support and motivation to achieve mutually negotiated goals" (Porter-O'Grady, 2003).

HEALTHCARE EVOLUTION

The evolution of healthcare over the past half century has increased the complexity of our systems. Over the past 50-plus years, great advances have occurred in almost every realm of healthcare. Haughom (2016) illustrates these changes when discussing the differences between healthcare in the 1960s and that of today. During this era, there were small private physician practices where the physician cared for patients in the office, making rounds within the acute care facility. The acute care facilities were smaller with less advanced capabilities, such as little modern imaging, primitive ICUs, lack of advanced anesthesia techniques, limited diagnostic techniques, and a lack of sophisticated catheterization procedures. There were also far fewer prescription medications, and the amount of published research was substantially less.

Essential Facts

The average life expectancy is 78 and 83 years of age for American men and women, respectively, with an average of 80 years of age for all Americans (World Population Review, 2019).

Today, we see large primary care practices with hospitalists caring for patients within very large, complex healthcare organizations comprising high-tech ICUs and numerous imaging and diagnostic abilities. Overall, healthcare professionals are faced with thousands of medications and exponentially expanded medical knowledge. In 2009, it was estimated that clinicians would need to read one article every 1.29 minutes to keep up to date on current information

Table 3.1

A Comparison of Healthcare Systems: The 1960s Versus Today

1960s Healthcare System	Today's Healthcare Systems
■ Small private physician practices with minimal staff ■ Physicians rounded in hospitals and knew all aspects of the patient	■ Large physician practices ■ Hospitalists care for acute care episodes ■ Many specialists and healthcare disciplines
■ Primitive ICUs ■ Telemetry	■ High-tech complex ICUs ■ Many monitoring capabilities

■ Few imaging abilities—primarily x-ray	■ Variety of available imaging:
	  a. CT scan
	  b. MRI
	  c. PET scans
	  d. EEGs, etc.

■ No advanced anesthesia techniques	■ Many anesthesia techniques and medications
■ Around 3-dozen medications	■ Thousands of medications
■ Small amount of literature	■ Exponentially expanded medical knowledge

(Haughom, 2016). These advances have led to not only increased complexity of the healthcare system but also increasing complexity of patient conditions. Technologic and medical advances in healthcare have permitted extended life expectancy, which is resulting in an increasing aging population of patients with multiple chronic conditions. All of these factors contribute to the complexity that is seen within healthcare systems today, which is outlined in Table 3.1.

CHAOS, COMPLEXITY, AND SYSTEMS THINKING

It is important for CNLs to understand how complexity affects the microsystem in which they work and lead. Complexity science emerged from Chaos theory and is the study of complex adaptive systems. Chaos theory was first utilized by scientists in fields such as mathematics, meteorology, and computer science (Kannampallil, Schauer, Cohen, & Patel, 2011). Scientific advances and computer capabilities provided scientists with the ability to develop high-level calculations on predictions of how certain systems would react. Their predictions were based on their belief that systems were predictable and behaved according to certain laws (Walsh, 2000). These predictions, however, resulted in completely different results from what was expected. The results proved that one could not always predict outcomes within complex systems, as the outcomes or results were sensitive to feedback from previously occurring events, and variations in feedback create even more significant alterations in outcomes (Walsh, 2000). The metaphor of the "butterfly effect" illustrates this thinking by suggesting that the flapping of a butterfly's wings in one part of the world can result in hurricanes in another part of the world from the change in air currents (Walsh, 2000). This same thinking can be used in our healthcare systems when looking at cause and effect as well as beginning change initiatives. Benson (2005) provides a great example of the butterfly effect when describing the implementation of overlay mattresses in a facility to reduce the incidence of pressure injuries. The mattress proved successful in decreasing pressure injuries, but the size, height, and slippery surface contributed to increased incidences of falls, which was an unexpected consequence.

Complexity and chaos thinking also allows us to see healthcare systems as nonlinear, unpredictable, and complex living and adaptive systems that live on the edge of chaos. It is at the "edge of chaos where change and creative ordering takes place through a dynamic, holistic, and reciprocal process" (Crowell, 2016, p. 23). These systems are seen as open systems possessing interconnected and interdependent elements that exchange energy, matter, and information. The interacting elements create feedback loops, which vary and influence the relationships between the elements, either positively or negatively. The interactions ultimately affect the workings of the entire system and are also considered unpredictable and unplanned, just as the previous discussion of the scientific predictions resulting in unpredictable outcomes. This unpredictability makes it very difficult or even impossible to predict specific outcomes. Consequently, when initiating change, nursing leaders must be constantly assessing and evaluating new initiatives to ensure results are proving to be positive, and negative consequences are recognized promptly.

Nonlinearity suggests that parts cannot be broken down. In linear systems, each part can be broken down, analyzed, and reconstructed to create a whole. This may be seen in a machine, as each piece of the machine can be broken down into parts and put back together. However, in nonlinear systems "the whole is more than the sum of its parts ... inputs are not proportional to outputs: a small (large) change in some variable or family of variables will not necessarily result in a small (large) change in the system" (Rickles, Hawe, & Shiell, 2007, p. 934). The inability to break components down into equal portions has to do with the "interrelationships between components" (Kannampallil et al., 2011, p. 944). The components are continuously interacting, causing variability in responses. This variability of responses is what contributes to the end product. An example of this can be seen when administering oxygen to a patient. It may seem a small intervention, but bodily processes interact differently in different people. Increasing oxygen levels in patients with chronic obstructive pulmonary disease may contribute to severe complications. In other situations, applying oxygen may improve oxygenation of the patient at the moment but may not be treating the underlying reason for the patient's compromised respiratory status. The Health Foundation (2010) states that "in its most simple form, complex adaptive systems is a way of thinking about and analyzing things by recognizing complexity, patterns, and interrelationships rather than focusing on cause and effect" (p. 6). Thus, when looking at patients and a healthcare organization's microsystem, you must focus on the interactions of people and systems to interpret how the interactions are affecting processes and outcomes.

So, why is it important for CNLs to consider complexity? When examining complex systems, the CNL must understand that predictions cannot always be made regarding interventions and change processes. Leaders must focus on interactions and relationships and not necessarily on steps and processes. Steps and processes often need to be changed during initiatives due to the interactions within the system. It is the interactions and relationships that inform leaders how the entity organizes and functions to achieve its outcomes. Nurse leaders must recognize how these systems interact in order to improve those interactions, which will create more positive feedback loops. For example, the ED is linked to a medical unit and most other microsystems within the healthcare system. How do interactions *within* the ED affect the microsystems of the organization? How do interactions *between* the ED and other microsystems affect one another and the whole of the organization?

A nurse working on a medical unit may not realize that their workflow may have a huge impact on the ED and the whole organization. We can see this sometimes with discharges, that is, when a nurse is behind in discharging a patient. What affect does this have on the ED and all the other different entities involved with that discharge? The patient may become upset if their discharge is delayed, and the family member transporting the patient may be impacted from being late in returning home to pick up their children from school. The ED is impacted because they are unable to transfer a patient out of an

ED bed to admit another patient from their waiting room. From one occurrence of a late discharge, the result may be that the ED's metrics decline due to the backup of patients in the waiting room, both the medical and ED patient satisfaction scores decline, and perhaps a seriously ill patient was not seen in time to save their life.

If we bring systems thinking into this scenario, we must focus on the interactions and on the relationships between the parts in order to understand the entity's organization, functioning, and outcomes. In the example of the late discharge, leaders must look at what organization and functioning of the parts led to the outcome of a late discharge and the effect on the system. Was the issue with the nurse who was too busy to tend to the discharge? If so, why was the nurse too busy? Was it the physician who did not write the order soon enough? Was it the lab that did not process the lab work in a timely manner in order to permit the physician to determine if the patient could be discharged? Was it the communication between professionals? The list could go on and on. Leaders must understand that negative events are usually the result of impediments in system processes and must look at all interactions to determine if the system has a flawed or broken piece or if one isolated incident led to the event. Again, what is the relationship between parts and interactions that have caused an interruption in processes?

Another example of complexity that affects CNLs and microsystems is the shortages of certain pharmaceutical products and supplies that have affected their ability to treat patients in a timely and effective manner. Shortages of medications require changes to be made by physicians in prescribing, possible pharmacy changes in obtaining alternative drug therapies, and nursing changes in order to obtain and maintain current knowledge of administration and side effects of substitute medications. Supply shortages such as IV tubing, saline solutions, and some devices may require the organization to find substitute devices, which may also require education of staff on how to correctly use the device. All of this also impacts the patients. This is an example of how organizations are also connected to outside entities that add to the complexity within the system.

Essential Facts

"Under circumstances where there is uncertainty about how to best deal with the situation, thinking outside the box and trying out different approaches is the most efficient strategy. In these cases, teams work as a CAS [complex adaptive system]" (Pype, Mertens, Helewaut , & Krystallidou, 2018, p. 8).

Table 3.2

Comparison of Organizational System Characteristics

Traditional Systems	Complex Adaptive Systems
Are mechanistic	Are living organisms
Are controlling and predictable	Are unpredictable
Are rigid, self-preserving	Are adaptive, flexible, creative
Behavior is controlled	Creativity is tapped
Find comfort in control	Embrace complexity
Recycle	Evolve continuously

When examining traditional systems versus complex adaptive systems, traditional systems are more mechanistic, are able to be controlled with predictable outcomes, are rigid with self-preserving behaviors, and their behaviors are recycled to achieve similar end products. These features coincide with manufacturing in that the systems are set up for employees to perform tasks toward completion of a product. In contrast, complex systems are living systems that have unpredictable workings and outcomes. However, the complex system is also flexible, with creativity of workers improving evolving processes. Members of complex systems embrace creativity and the complexity that goes along with it to continuously advance processes and care. Healthcare is a complex adaptive system, in that care is provided to complex patients, and each member of the care team brings their own knowledge, ideas, creativity, and behaviors to work to care for patients in individualized manners (Table 3.2). It is essential that leaders recognize these differences when leading microsystems and teams. Leading also requires one to look at whom they are leading. Just as systems have changed over the years, workers have also changed, which requires not only an understanding of leadership principles but also the differences in workers to truly understand how to lead.

KNOWLEDGE WORKERS

As noted previously, many changes have occurred within healthcare and healthcare settings over the years that affect our systems today. Changes have also occurred that affect the workers within these organizations. In the past, many hospitals had their own schools of nursing that educated students to work within the hospital setting. As greater advances in healthcare and the profession occurred, education moved to academic settings. These changes have contributed to higher levels of knowledge of the workers and a difference in how they view the workplace. According to Porter-O'Grady & Malloch (2018), movement of training outside of the work environment has contributed to workers feeling a decreased sense of responsibility to the organization. Therefore, the organization no longer owns the workers, and workers are no longer indebted to the organization for their training and knowledge. Workers have more of a choice in where they work, and organizations are now competing for the knowledge that workers bring with them (Porter-O'Grady & Malloch, 2018).

Essential Facts

Millennial nurses are less concerned about organizational loyalty and more interested in helping others, personal engagement, job security, and good compensation benefits (Hampton & Welsh, 2019).

It is this knowledge that leaders must embrace and harness to improve systems and work processes. There is greater value of workers today, and that value comes from the knowledge they hold. Organizations must recognize that they need the knowledge the worker holds more than the worker needs one particular organization (Porter-O'Grady, 2003). Therefore, leaders must not only lead, but they must lead by developing relationships with employees to permit the workers to feel valued and appreciated. Consequently, leading in today's healthcare systems requires an understanding of the changes and characteristics of organizations as well as employees. Leadership styles of the past may not be good enough to move microsystems and healthcare organizations forward in today's complex environments.

TRADITIONAL LEADERSHIP

Leadership traits and qualities have evolved over time similarly to how healthcare has evolved. Leadership developed throughout the rise of industry and changed and advanced as industry developed. Early on, leaders were charged with maintaining control of the workforce in order to get the job or task done quickly and efficiently. This was mostly done to stay ahead of the competition. Leaders in this era were charged with directing activities, controlling processes, and evaluating end products. Several leadership styles developed throughout this time and remain in use in many organizations today. The most common of these styles include bureaucratic or authoritarian, democratic, laissez-faire, and transactional. These styles may be effective for CNLs to utilize in some situations.

In authoritarian leadership, the leader makes all the decisions without considering input from others. To enforce rules, negative reinforcement and punishment are used (Frandsen, 2014). This leadership style does not tolerate mistakes, and blame is placed upon individuals. Results are well-defined group actions that are usually predictable, which may provide a sense of security to members. This style may be effective during times of crises.

Characteristics of authoritarian style of leadership include the following:

a. Maintains strong control
b. Motivates others by coercion
c. Directs others with commands
d. Downward communication flow
e. Decision-making does not include others
f. Criticism is punitive (Frandsen, 2014)

Democratic leadership can be used when attempting to engage staff members or when working within teams. It is considered a shared leadership model where team members are welcomed to share ideas and input. The leader provides guidance and is less likely to mandate processes. Leaders utilizing this style must be cautious in ensuring roles are defined and order is maintained. Democratic leaders may come across as indecisive, so effective communication is essential.

Characteristics of democratic leaders include the following:

a. Maintains less control
b. Communication flows up and down
c. Emphasis is on the group rather than the leader
d. Criticism is constructive
e. Decision-making is a team effort

Laissez-faire leadership style takes a hands-off approach and provides little or no direction or supervision. Because the leader is so disengaged, changes rarely occur, decisions are not made, and any quality improvement is a reactive approach instead of being a proactive approach (Frandsen, 2014).

Characteristics of laissez-faire leaders include the following:

a. Permissiveness with little or no control
b. Motivation by support when requested by the group or individuals

c. Little or no direction
d. Communication flows upward and downward
e. Decision-making is dispersed throughout the group
f. Emphasis on the group
g. Criticism withheld (Frandsen 2014)

Transactional leaders use a task-oriented approach. When given a task, a person is expected to do what is assigned. This may be effective when dealing with emergency situations, but if used on a daily basis, staff tend to focus on tasks instead of looking at the entire patient or process. Transactional leaders operate by the principle of management by exception; if everything is status quo, the leader will not intervene (Giltinane, 2013).

Characteristics of transactional leaders include the following:

a. Focuses on reward and punishment
b. Emphasis placed on completion of tasks
c. Criticism is punitive
d. Downward communication

Transformational leadership is a newer form of leadership that was developed by James MacGregor Burns in 1978. Burns (1978) proposed there was a difference between management and leadership, suggesting leaders assisted followers in moving forward through building morale and motivation. Transformational leaders lead by exemplifying values and inspiring others to achieve a shared mission and goals. Leaders are said to inspire and motivate others through exemplifying behaviors and attitudes that inspire others to trust, admire, and exhibit loyalty toward the leader (Grossman & Valiga, 2017).

Characteristics of transformational leadership include the following:

a. Motivationally inspire others
b. Consider individual contributions
c. Provide intellectual stimulation
d. Inspires others to follow mission/vision (Grossman & Valiga, 2017)

As you can see, differences in leadership approaches coincide with organizational environments (Table 3.3). Organizations evolved from the industrial/mechanistic environments where the object was to produce products in an efficient, timely manner. Everything was to be outlined and planned down to the smallest detail. The expectation was that by planning future activities with great specificity, an organization could respond to the current situation accurately and effectively. The idea of planning assumes much more control over circumstances. Leaders were charged with maintaining order and ensuring workers were producing. Innovations came from the top, not from the workers. The workers were told what to do, and they had to comply.

You may still see many of these leadership models being used today; however, they are not always relevant for sustaining leadership and change within our systems.

LEADERSHIP WITHIN COMPLEX ENVIRONMENTS

Leading within complex settings requires new ideas in the way of leadership to guide others' actions in creating positive results, instead of demanding particular actions. Today's workers are not assembly line workers who follow strict rules; they are knowledge workers who have the knowledge and ability to think and develop new ways of performing care. Leaders must harness this knowledge by empowering workers to share their knowledge, adding to the knowledge of others as well as the organization as a whole. Giltinane (2013) discusses how leaders should lead to develop "shared values, vision and expectations to enhance their organization's planned goals and overall effectiveness" (p. 35).

Leaders in today's healthcare systems must distance themselves from mechanistic ways of leading and attempt to bring teams and groups together to effectively embrace change (The Health Foundation, 2010). Leading in this type of environment requires individuals to utilize complexity leadership principles. These principles include knowledge of complexity science, leading by using a transformational style that is collaborative, self-reflective, and relationship based (Crowell, 2016). Weberg (2017) states that complexity leaders must also be adaptive and dynamic, which requires leaders to consider diversity of opinions from others within the environment. Relationships are developed, and an importance is placed on sustaining relationships and how these relationships self-regulate and organize throughout time and change (Crowell, 2016).

Relationship development is important as one cannot lead without having followers. Leaders need to understand that people will only follow if the leader possesses skills and traits that make people want to follow. Leaders must genuinely care for the people they lead, demonstrating respect for each member while creating a feeling of excitement for change (Grossman & Valiga, 2017). Therefore, leaders must create environments that empower workers, permitting them to feel they are a valued part of the mission of the organization. Leaders must utilize effective communication, which is essential for leaders to convey an honest interest in the thoughts, feelings, and knowledge that colleagues bring to the work environment. Development of these skills and traits enhances the development of leader–follower relationships within a complex environment.

Essential Facts

> CNLs lead at the point of care, providing opportunities to interact with all of the healthcare team members. Joining staff as a colleague within their work environment respects their time, increasing engagement.

CNLs are considered authentic leaders who lead horizontally where the leader's influence is earned through knowledge, education, and respect (Monaghan & Swihart, 2010). CNLs use a horizontal

Table 3.3

Comparison of Leader Characteristics in Complex Adaptive Systems and Traditional Systems

Complex Adaptive Systems	Traditional Systems
Are open, responsive, catalytic	Are controlling, mechanistic
Offer alternatives	Repeat the past
Are collaborative, engaging others	Are in charge
Are connected	Are autonomous
Are adaptable	Are self-preserving
Realize change is inevitable	Resist change, bury contradictions
Are engaged, change is continuously emerging	Are disengaged, nothing ever changes
Value persons	Value position, structures
Shift as processes unfold	Hold formal position
Help others	Set rules
Allow others to help with decision-making	Make decisions
Are listeners	Are knowers
Recognize importance of followers	Downplay role of followers

leadership approach in their practice as they do not have formal positional authority over the staff. However, the CNL is still able to exert influence in their microsystem through changing plans of care, delegating and supervising the care given, and by delivering and managing improvements in patient safety and clinical outcomes (Monaghan & Swihart, 2010). This is all accomplished through the use of effective leadership skills that coincide with the complexity of the environment. Therefore, it is essential that CNLs have an understanding of complexity thinking and leadership to move teams and processes forward.

Moving forward as complexity leaders, CNLs will have certain challenges within chaotic/complex environments. This will require the CNL to embrace change and the circumstances surrounding that change while sorting out their implications and applications. Leaders will need to be able to identify what type of change is needed and how to implement those changes. Leaders will also need to develop a regard for risk taking and for the boundaries of understanding that risk. They must take smaller steps and identify the consequences of each step to determine if it is the best direction to move forward. Technological advances, along with the need and capacity to adapt to them, are not going to go away. These advances bring exceptional possibilities, but they also bring further mountains to climb. Leaders will be called upon to teach coping and adaptation skills, learn new skills, and apply them in new ways in new settings. It is hard to imagine what the healthcare system will be like in 20 years.

These are all of the ideals of the complexity leader, which coincide perfectly with the ideals and beliefs of the CNL being a clinician, outcomes manager, client advocate, educator, information manager, systems analyst, team manager member of a profession, and lifelong learner.

Clinical Nurse Leader Vignette 3.1:
CNL Leadership: Improving the Onboarding Experience and Reducing Turnover Rates in a Hematologic Oncology Unit

A hematologic oncology unit was concerned with high turnover rates of new graduate nurses. Jill, the CNL on the unit, assessed the issue and determined that a major problem was a knowledge gap in caring for the specific disease processes of the population. Nurses often worked on the unit for 6 months to a year before they were able to take specific oncology courses offered by the organization. This

> *often resulted in new nurses feeling unprepared and unskilled in their work, decreasing self-confidence and overall satisfaction for their work. Jill used her knowledge of complexity and transformational leadership in attempting to increase support by fostering relationships and trust during the first 6 months of the nurses' employment. Jill developed a structured residency program for the new graduates that included disease specific education, scheduled relationship building meetings, and provided mentors to assist the nurses during their transition to practice. The early educational sessions, which focused on the specific patient population, expanded clinical knowledge of disease processes, and enhanced the nurses' critical thinking skills. The regularly scheduled meetings and mentors fostered the development of trust and belonging as relationships were developed. The program ultimately improved the new nurses' onboarding experience, decreased turnover of staff saving the unit thousands of dollars, and improved the care of the patient.*

References

Benson, H. (2005). Chaos and complexity: Applications for healthcare quality and patient safety. *Journal for Healthcare Quality, 27*(5), 4–10.

Burns, J. M. (1978). *Leadership*. New York, NY: Harper and Row.

Crowell, D. (2016). *Complexity leadership nursing's role in health-care delivery* (2nd ed.). Philadelphia, PA: F.A. Davis Company.

Frandsen, B. (2014). *Nursing leadership management and leadership styles*. Retrieved from American Association of Nurse Assessment Coordination: https://www.aanac.org/docs/white-papers/2013-nursing-leadership---management-leadership-styles.pdf?sfvrsn=4

Giltinane, C. (2013). Leadership styles and theories. *Nursing Standard, 27*(41), 35–39. doi:10.7748/ns2013.06.27.41.35.e7565

Grossman, S., & Valiga, T. M. (2017). *The new leadership challenge creating the future of nursing* (5th ed.). Philadelphia, PA: F.A. Davis Company.

Hampton, D., & Welsh, D. (2019). Work values of generation Z nurses. *Journal of Nursing Administration, 49*(10), 480–486. doi:10.1097/NNA.0000000000000791

Haughom, J. (2016, February 9). *Healthcare quality, safety, and complexity: The challenging trio* [Video file]. Retrieved from https://www.youtube.com/watch?v=AXD-iInmLVE

The Health Foundation. (2010). *Evidence scan: Complex adaptive systems*. Retrieved from https://www.health.org.uk/publications/complex-adaptive-systems

Kannampallil, T. G., Schauer, G. F., Cohen, T., & Patel, V. L. (2011). Considering complexity in healthcare systems. *Journal of Biomedical Informatics, 44*(6), 943–947. doi:10.1016/j.jbi.2011.06.006

Monaghan, H., & Swihart, D. (2010). *Clinical nurse leader: Transforming practice, transforming care. A model for the clinician at the point of care.* Sarasota, FL: Visioning HealthCare Inc.

Porter-O'Grady, T. (2003). A different age for leadership part 1: New context, new content. *Journal of Nursing Administration, 33*(2), 105–110. doi:10.1097/00005110-200302000-00007

Porter-O'Grady, T., & Malloch, K. (2018). *Quantum leadership creating sustainable value in healthcare.* Burlington, MA: Jones and Bartlett Learning.

Pype, P., Mertens, F., Helewaut, F., & Krystallidou, D. (2018). Healthcare teams as complex adaptive systems: Understanding team behaviour through team members' perception of interpersonal interaction. *BMC Health Services Research, 18*(1), 570. doi:10.1186/s12913-018-3392-3

Rickles, D., Hawe, P., & Shiell, A. (2007). A simple guide to chaos and complexity. *Journal of Epidemiology and Community, 61*(11), 933–937. doi:10.1136/jech.2006.054254

Weberg, D. (2017). Innovation leadership behaviors: Starting the complexity journey. In S. Davidson, D. Weberg, T. Porter-O'Grady, & K. Malloch (Eds.), *Leadership for evidence-based innovation in nursing and health professions* (pp. 43–76). Burlington, MA: Jones and Bartlett Learning.

World Population Review. (2019). *United States population 2019.* Retrieved from https://worldpopulationreview.com/countries/united-states-population/

4

Microsystem Assessment and the 5Ps

Ann Deerhake

Everyone is a genius. But if you judge a fish on its ability to climb a tree, it will live its whole life believing it is stupid.
~Albert Einstein

INTRODUCTION

Courtesy of your education and hard work, you have the tools to establish yourself as a leader. You are prepared to encourage followers to work alongside you in an effort to improve care within your shared workplace. Additionally, in previous chapters, the initial framework to promote the clinical nurse leader (CNL) role, move into CNL practice, and lead within a microsystem was presented. Now, we take the first step toward actually creating change within your microsystem by refreshing your skills regarding microsystem assessment. Every healthcare setting has strengths and weaknesses; your role as a CNL is to identify these, looking for holes in systems and risks to patients, all the while being realistic regarding the purpose of your microsystem and nonjudgmental of those who work there. Utilizing the 5P framework to assess your microsystem is a reasonable place to start. This chapter provides a quick reference on performing a microsystem assessment in various healthcare settings, highlighting the 5Ps, including purpose, patients, professionals, processes, and patterns.

After reading this chapter, you will be able to:

1. Identify quality issues within your microsystem
2. Recognize the impact of barriers when working to improve your microsystem
3. Differentiate assessment techniques within multiple healthcare settings
4. Assess your microsystem by applying the 5P framework.

WHY DO CNLs ASSESS?

Essential Facts

"The main idea (of microsystem assessment) is for the microsystem to build understanding and to discover its capability from the inside out" (Nelson, Batalden, & Godfrey, 2007, p. 260).

According to Chaos theory, "the whole is more than the sum of its parts" (Rickles, Hawe, & Shiell, 2007, p. 934). In harmony with this idea, the vision for the CNL role is based upon being a bedside generalist who works to find and repair issues within our ailing healthcare system, one microsystem at a time, in the hopes the end result will be high-performing microsystems and even more superior macrosystems. In most healthcare settings, CNLs do not specialize in specific patient populations or diagnoses; however, they certainly do become clinical experts regarding their particular microsystem. For this reason, CNLs are specifically educated and perfectly positioned to conduct thorough assessments of their workplaces, discovering issues within interprofessional teams, gaps in care delivery, and risks to patients.

Problem Identification

As the CNL clinically in charge of a particular microsystem, you are responsible to be cognizant and curious regarding the activity within your unit. Every microsystem has issues requiring attention, regardless of the setting. As an outsider looking in, it can be quite easy to see areas needing improvement; however, it is easy to question yourself, asking "Is this just how things are done here?" According to organizational culture expert Edgar Schein (2017), "different people have different biases and assumptions about what is important," which can contribute to lack of common goals among employees (p. 1). Processes within microsystems are an integral part of its function and purpose; proposing change can bring forth support and agreement, as well as controversy and conflict. However, opening discussion about process improvement is crucial to the health of a microsystem because it allows for others to voice concerns, many times bringing forth additional, less apparent issues that may contribute to the root cause of more visible problems. Scheduling formal and initiating impromptu conversations with frontline, managerial, and administrative staff is the best way to determine and prioritize issues.

Talking with frontline staff regarding their views in relation to unit problems is a great place to start when attempting to discover process issues. If you have developed rapport with those working within your microsystem, this should already be a common occurrence. Utilizing active listening techniques when attending meetings and educational offerings within the microsystem will help you determine problems and identify specific stakeholders you might consider approaching to garner more information. Less formal but perhaps even more effective discovery methods include sharing meals as well as assisting and rounding within the microsystem. Meeting staff where the majority of their work takes place shows that you value both their time and input. Additionally, as the staff begin to understand the function of the CNL role by watching you work, they will approach you more frequently about issues that concern them and their patients.

Microsystem nursing managers frequently have already determined microsystem problems based on feedback from frontline staff and directives from administrative staff. Many times, managers will informally approach CNLs with a punch list of clinical items needing work. The reason for this is twofold; managers (a) are well aware of both metric-based and non-metric-based deficiencies within their microsystem and (b) wish to delegate time-consuming quality improvement activities to those who can successfully conduct them. Simply put, microsystem managers are inundated with data regarding the function and productivity of their unit and require assistance in clinical process improvement. Keep in mind, however, that most managers consider themselves the final decision-makers within their microsystem, and working in conjunction with them is a major strategy toward CNL and microsystem success. Similar to building rapport with frontline staff, working to hone the CNL–manager relationship is critical. Scheduling a weekly huddle with your microsystem manager is a great way to keep communication flowing as well as educate unfamiliar managers with the CNL role. Delineating between managerial and CNL microsystem tasks is absolutely necessary.

Administrators within organizations have set metric-based goals they, and you as their subordinate, work hard to achieve. Frequently, successfully attaining these goals is linked to financial incentives for the organization, revealing an important reason why the CNL role was initiated in healthcare. As said in *To Err Is Human: Building a Safer Health System* (National Academy of Sciences, 1999), the cost of preventable medical mistakes lies somewhere between $17 billion and $29 billion. Rodziewicz and Hipskind (2019) suggest that healthcare-related infections may account for a $35 billion increase to annual U.S. healthcare expenditures. Although we may not always understand or agree with how organizations prioritize problems, it is clear they have a large burden to shoulder when it comes to healthcare costs. As information managers, we need to take these issues back to the bedside and work on creative solutions to align microsystem patient goals with macrosystem financial goals; if we can do both, everyone wins. As an example, Table 4.1 displays the financial impact that CNLs had on a 637-bed tertiary care facility and community hospital located in the Northeastern United States, all the while improving patient outcomes (Wilson et al., 2013).

Barriers to Solving Problems

Issues that exist within microsystems many times are part of the microsystem culture, making changes to these issues, even when they are beneficial for all, extremely difficult. Schein (2017) states "think of culture as being for the group or organization what personality or character is to the individual" (loc. 6274). How difficult is it for people to change their personality or character? Incredibly hard, because personality and character are part of who they are as a person. For microsystems, culture is part of the reason they exist, and they frequently define themselves based on culture. The processes and workflows currently in place are part of the microsystem culture. For instance, if you ask bedside ICU nurses to change their

Table 4.1

Financial Outcomes Attributable to Clinical Nurse Leadership in a 637-Bed Tertiary Care Facility and Community Hospital in the Northeastern United States

Intervention	Outcome Measure	Interval (months)	Savings (U.S. Dollars)
Elimination of autotransfusion in total knee replacement patients	Costs related to a decrease in equipment and staff time	12	$150,000
Long-term ventilator rounds	Costs related to decreased ventilator days	60	$1,000,000
Postoperative craniotomy pathway	Costs related to decreased LOS	9	$170,000
Postprocedure myelogram pathway	Costs related to decreased postprocedure LOS	12	$139,000
Total knee replacement: implementation of femoral block	Costs related to decreased recovery room and hospital LOS	12	$1,200,000
		Total	$2,659,000

LOS, length of stay.

Source: Wilson, L., Orff, S., Gerry, T., Shirley, B. R., Tabor, D., Caiazzo, K., & Rouleau, D. (2013). Evolution of an innovative role: The clinical nurse leader. *Journal of Nursing Management, 21*(1), 175–181. doi:10.1111/j.1365-2834.2012.01454.x, p. 179.

workflow to accommodate an additional patient population or diagnosis, you might meet with resistance. with responses such as: "We're an ICU! We don't take telemetry patients," or if you propose primary care nurses begin making postvisit follow-up phone calls to patients, you might hear, "Usually patients call us; we don't call them." Solving quality problems means creating an adapted cultural identity for your microsystem.

Adaptation of microsystem identity can be a difficult, lengthy process that can be hard to do and sustain. Providing staff with the rationale behind your actions, as well as opportunities to get involved, encourages ownership of the proposed change, rather than simply buy-in. Building a transdisciplinary transformation team comprising microsystem professionals who embrace and understand the need for change is key. Rather than simply coming together with other disciplines, taking a transdisciplinary approach means encouraging team members to learn and understand other disciplines' workflows and factor them into decision-making. Regardless of how or where you choose to begin this journey toward microsystem change, the first step in developing a reasonable quality improvement plan is completing a thorough microsystem assessment.

MICROSYSTEM ASSESSMENT IN DIFFERENT SETTINGS

Within the early days of CNL practice, Nelson, Batalden, and Godfrey (2007) discussed the importance of following a specific procedure when assessing clinical microsystems, proposing the utilization of the 5P framework. Within this context, CNLs can assess the purpose, patients, professionals, processes, and patterns of a given microsystem (p. 258). McKeon et al. (2009) further defined this approach, suggesting:

> *Structure* involves how the microsystem is organized, operates, and relates to other microsystems, leadership roles, reporting mechanisms, macroorganizational support, resource allocation (human, financial, supplies/equipment), and information technology. *Process* involves the culture of the microsystem, how care is delivered and by whom, the interdependence of the interdisciplinary team, case mix of providers, hours worked by staff, populations of patients, health outcomes, and process improvement activities. *Pattern* involves communication within, among, and across disciplines and microsystems, relationships among interdisciplinary teams, clinical outcomes, delays in provision of care, risk, and potential error. (p. 374)

How you choose to examine your microsystem is strictly up to you, keeping in mind that conducting a complete yet concise microsystem assessment is time well spent, because it will guide you toward effective CNL practice and your microsystem toward excellence. For this book, we will be utilizing the 5P assessment recommended by Nelson, Batalden, and Godfrey as well as their free assessment tools, retrieved from the *Microsystem Academy Knowledge Center* at http://clinicalmicrosystem.org.

Purpose

The operative question here is, "Why do we exist?" (Exhibit 4.1). For those around us, what purpose do we serve? Opening these questions up for discussion can be a useful exercise as well as an enlightening

Exhibit 4.1

The Purpose Portion of the Inpatient Unit Profile 5P Assessment Template

A. Purpose:
Why does your unit exist?

	Site Contact:	Date:
Administrative Director:	Nurse Director:	Medical Director:

Source: The Dartmouth Institute Microsystem Academy, Godfrey, M., Nelson, E., & Batalden, P.; Institute of Medicine. (2005). *Microsystem Academy Knowledge Center: Inpatient Workbook* (p. 6). Retrieved from http://clinicalmicrosystem.org/knowledge-center/workbooks/.

experience for all. Most microsystem employees have an idea of their purpose but have never really spent time pondering the idea. Mission statements can reflect a microsystem's purpose, yet many times they are less than specific (Nelson, Batalden, & Godfrey, 2007). You may be surprised at the different ideas and priorities that others bring forth.

Essential Facts

The CNL was designed to be versatile, with a skill set that can be applied in any healthcare setting (L'Ecuyer, Shatto, Hoffmann, & Crecelius, 2016).

Within primary care settings, functions will vary; however, the basic purposes are similar. According to the American Academy of Family Physicians (AAFP; 2019), primary care practices are a patient's initial "point of entry into the healthcare system and [serve] as the continuing focal point for all needed healthcare services" (AAFP, para 5). This healthcare home, as the name implies, provides patients with comfort, consistency, and security. Healthcare consumers look to primary care providers as medical confidantes, keepers of information, and coordinators of medical care. This is where patients go to get help for managing chronic disease or advice for working toward optimal health and wellness.

Ambulatory care units, whether for emergency, urgent, or scheduled care, provide varied yet specific services to patients. Healthcare consumers seek ED assistance for immediate needs, trusting they will receive the diagnosis and treatment they require efficiently and expediently. Urgent care centers are an extension of both primary care and emergency settings, providing care when physician offices are closed, treating less critical patients than EDs, and reducing delays in treatment during evening and weekend hours. Outpatient departments deliver a multitude of services including preventive screenings, diagnostic procedures, infusion and wound services.

The purpose of acute care settings is temporary in nature for most patients. They provide for patients during acute illness, helping them either return home in a better state of health or move toward a peaceful death within the hospital or at home. Hospitals also take a keen interest in assisting families and caregivers to care for their loved ones. Additionally, acute care facilities provide care for well patients such as mothers, newborns, and elective surgery candidates. It is easy to surmise that different units within acute care facilities will have different purposes; fully taking into account the need that each microsystem fulfills is important.

Long-term care organizations provide an alternate home for those in need. Much like primary care settings, extended care facilities can help residents work toward managing chronic disease as well as promoting wellness. They also assist patients with temporary rehabilitation, skilled care, and terminal conditions. Differing from primary care settings, microsystems within extended care facilities will have purposes based on the type of care needed by and delivered to patients.

Patients

Nelson, Batalden, and Godfrey (2007) state "patients have valuable insight into the quality and process of care health professionals provide" (p. 396). The questions to ask yourself here are "What are the most common populations seen within this microsystem?" and "How do we group them to give care?" (Exhibit 4.2). For example, in an outpatient unit, do we group populations by those who receive infusions versus those who receive wound care? Or do we group them by diagnoses or time required for care? Or do we perhaps do both? However we choose to answer these questions, it is important we understand that those who work within microsystems possess knowledge regarding the specific patient populations they serve (Nelson, Batalden, & Godfrey, 2007). This makes complete sense; after all, these healthcare workers are delivering care daily to them. However, not all members of a microsystem will have the same view of the unit's patient mix because of varying roles as well as different days and shifts worked by employees. Starting these conversations with staff will likely provide insight for all.

Exhibit 4.2

The Patient Portion of the Inpatient Unit Profile 5P Assessment Template

B. Know Your Patients: Take a close look into your unit and create a "high-level" picture of the PATIENT POPULATION that you serve. Who are they? What resources do they use? How do the patients view the care they receive?

Est. Age Distribution of Pts.:	%	List Your Top 10 Diagnoses/Conditions	Pt. Satisfaction Scores	% Always
19–50 years		1. 6.	Nurses	
51–65 years		2. 7.	Doctors	
66–75 years		3. 8.	Environment	
76+ years		4. 9.	Pain	
		5. 10.	Discharge	% Yes
% Females			Overall	% Excellent
Living Situation	**%**	**Point of Entry**	**% Pt. Population Census: Do These Numbers Change by Season? (Y/N)**	**Y/N**
Married		Admissions	Pt. Census by Hour	
Domestic Partner		Clinic	Pt. Census by Day	
Live Alone		ED	Pt. Census by Week	
Live With Others		Transfer	Pt. Census by Year	
Skilled Nursing Facility		**Discharge Disposition**	% 30-Day Readmit Rate	

(continued)

Exhibit 4.2.

The Patient Portion of the Inpatient Unit Profile 5P Assessment Template (*continued*)

Living Situation	%	Point of Entry	%	Pt. Population Census: Do These Numbers Change by Season? (Y/N)	Y/N
Nursing Home		Home		Our Patients in Other Units	
Homeless		Home With Visiting Nurse		Off Service Patients on Our Unit	
Patient Type	**LOS Avg.** Range	Skilled Nursing Facility		Frequency of Inability to Admit Pt.	
Medical		Other Hospital		*Complete "Through the Eyes of Your Patient," p. 8	
Surgical		Rehab Facility			
Mortality Rate		Transfer to ICU			

Source: The Dartmouth Institute Microsystem Academy; Godfrey, M. Nelson, E., & Batalden, P.; Institute of Medicine. (2005). *Microsystem Academy Knowledge Center: Inpatient Workbook* (p. 6). Retrieved from http://clinicalmicrosystem.org/knowledge-center/workbooks/.

Essential Facts

Clinical nurse leaders have improved the culture of caring by developing relationships with patients that can increase patient satisfaction and outcomes (L'Ecuyer, Shatto, Hoffmann, & Crecelius, 2016).

In primary care settings, it is important to consider how much is known about each individual patient, including which social determinants of health (SDH) are most influential when making care decisions. Asking patients questions regarding, but not limited to, socioeconomic status, communication preferences, religious beliefs, cultural influences, and knowledge of disease/treatment may help to individualize care, increasing effectiveness. Points to discuss with frontline staff might include the following: What types of patients do we see at what time of year? Are there common diagnoses we see all year round? What are the most common chronic health problems that patients possess? Do we treat well patients or only ill patients? Staff discussions and meetings will undoubtedly bring forth more questions regarding patient types cared for within the practice. Compiling this information into a database can help CNLs monitor patient risks and outcomes, as well as patient and staff educational/informational needs.

According to the American Society of Healthcare Engineering (ASHE; 2017), ambulatory care is delivered in a variety of ways, including "Internet platforms ... mobile care ... retail clinics ... urgent care ... freestanding emergency departments ... work clinics ... primary care clinics ... specialty care centers" ("Design considerations," para. 7–15). They continue, stating patients may be transactional, meaning they have one focus, such as seeking diagnosis of a fracture or administration of a vaccination. Conversely, they may be multidimensional, meaning they require a more overall assessment of needs, such as those patients receiving infusions or psychiatric treatment. Additionally, ambulatory care patients can visit homogeneous settings such as procedurally oriented endoscopy centers; heterogeneous settings such as general outpatient clinics; or combination settings such as clinics providing both wound care and IV antibiotic infusions. What does this all mean? Assessing the patient population in ambulatory microsystems is extremely variable, yet very specific to your particular microsystem. Determining the most common diagnoses of patients frequenting your ambulatory setting requires review of purpose, scheduling, care delivery, and patient outcomes.

Again, depending on the type of ambulatory setting you are assessing, looking at the SDH influence on each patient is important.

Microsystems within acute care can also have patients with similar or variable diagnoses, such as within an obstetrics unit versus a medical–surgical unit. Patients in the perioperative setting, while similar in that they are all presenting for surgery, have a multitude of diagnoses and required procedures. Furthermore, within the acute care setting, it is necessary to consider patients' families and significant others to be on the receiving end of care, especially in critical care areas. McKeon et al. (2009) posit the importance of "analyz(ing) the microsystem's ability to promote patient and family participation in care," especially focusing on "dignity and respect" (p. 376). Identifying the most common patient diagnoses and treatments within your microsystem, as well as the physical, educational, and emotional support needed by patients and families, is the best place to start when assessing the patient population within your unit.

Long-term care facilities house both well residents requiring minimal assistance and sick patients needing complete care, as well as everyone in between. Depending on where your microsystem exists within the long-term care system, your patients will vary. Group homes, skilled nursing, assisted living, and independent living units many times exist on the same campus, allowing for specific microsystems to evolve and movement of patients between units. Some patients have chronic disease or cognitive dysfunction, many times exacerbated by acute episodes of illness, while others may simply have mobility issues. Perhaps the most important part of patient assessment within a long-term care microsystem is understanding that most patients and families chose to move to this type of setting as a permanent home. According to Halfon et al, it is important to "anticipate(s) the risks and future (patient) needs in order to restore baseline independence and function" (as cited in Rankin, Ralyea, & Sotomayor, 2018, p. 270).

Professionals

According to Nelson, Batalden, and Godfrey (2007), "creating a joyful work environment starts with a basic understanding of staff perceptions of the practice" (p. 402). Staff working in primary care may include physicians, nurse practitioners, physician assistants, nurses, nursing assistants, medical assistants, schedulers, and secretaries. While the primary care setting may include only a few different disciplines, an important part of their role is to coordinate with consulting physicians, laboratory and radiology professionals, pharmacy staff, rehabilitation therapists, and insurance company personnel.

Some practices have these ancillary professionals on site, whereas others contract out for services. Another factor to consider is the organizational structure beyond the primary care microsystem, as many provider practices are now part of larger medical groups. For these types of primary care settings, many decisions for the microsystem are made at the corporate level. Getting to know the structure of your microsystem is critical (Exhibit 4.3).

Essential Facts

"The goal is to have the right person doing the right thing at the right time" (The Dartmouth Institute Microsystem Academy, Godfrey, Nelson, & Batalden; Institute of Medicine, 2005, p. 406).

Professionals within the ambulatory care setting will vary depending on the type of care provided by the site. The common link, however, is that providers are constantly present at most ambulatory care settings during hours of operation. For example, freestanding EDs and urgent care centers always have a provider on duty; patients know that they will see a physician, nurse practitioner, or physician's assistant when they enter the building. Retail clinics also always have a provider present as well; however, support staff can vary across settings. A more technologically savvy offering, online video visits, delivers a provider directly to the patient's computer or smart phone. Identifying professionals working within these types of settings may be more difficult, given the transient nature of the care provided and the possible need for consults and transfers. It is important to note that within all of these settings, relationships exist between the ambulatory care center and higher levels of care, adding to the list of professionals working in the microsystem.

Generally, acute care microsystems can include a myriad of disciplines, depending on their purpose and type of care delivered. For example, a perioperative setting could include general surgeons, specialty surgeons, physician assistants, anesthesiologists, nurse anesthetists, perfusionists, surgical nurses, surgical techs, pharmacists, laboratory staff, and radiology personnel. Additionally, representatives from a variety of equipment suppliers may be present on any given day for technology support. Other acute care microsystems may consist of considerably less personnel, all the while working closely with ancillary departments such as the laboratory, radiology, and rehabilitation therapy departments. Also, telemedicine has increased the availability of specialist care, adding to the microsystem's care

Exhibit 4.3

The Professionals Portion of the Inpatient Unit Profile 5P Assessment Template

C. *Know Your Professionals:* Use the following template to create a comprehensive picture of your unit. Who does what and when? Is the right person doing the right activity? Are roles being optimized? Are all roles who contribute to the patient experience listed?

Current Staff	Day FTEs	Evening FTEs	Night FTEs	Weekend FTEs	Over-Time by Role	Admitting Medical Service	%
MD Total						Internal Medicine	
Hospitalists Total						Hematology/Oncology	
Unit Leader Total						Pulmonary	
CNSs Total						Family Practice	
RNs Total						ICU	
LPNs Total						Other	
LNAs Total						**Supporting Diagnostic Departments**	
Residents Total							
Technicians Total						(e.g., Respiratory, Lab, Cardiology, Pulmonary, Radiology)	
Secretaries Total							
Clinical Resource Coord.							

Social Worker

Health Service Assts.

Ancillary Staff

Do you use Per Diems? _____ Yes _____ No

Do you use Travelers? _____ Yes _____ No

Do you use On-Call Staff? _____ Yes _____ No

Do you use a Float Pool? _____ Yes _____ No

Staff Satisfaction Scores		%
How stressful is the unit?	% Not Satisfied	
Would you recommend it as a good place to work?	% Strongly Agree	

*Each staff member should complete the Personal Skills Assessment and "The Activity Survey", pp. 10–12

Source: The Dartmouth Institute Microsystem Academy, Godfrey, M., Nelson, E., & Batalden, P.; Institute of Medicine. (2005). *Microsystem Academy Knowledge Center: Inpatient Workbook* (p. 6). Retrieved from http://clinicalmicrosystem.org/knowledge-center/workbooks/.

options. An inpatient neurological unit may consist of round-the-clock care delivered by nurses, nursing assistants, and secretaries, with visits from physicians, nurse practitioners, clinical nurse specialists, physician assistants, case managers, pharmacists, dieticians, respiratory, and rehabilitation therapists sporadically. Many acute care microsystems do not have providers routinely present, utilizing nursing staff to be the primary care givers as well as the eyes and ears of the providers. Hospitals also frequently offer additional services such as financial counseling, complementary alternative medicine, pet therapy, and spiritual care. When assessing professionals in the acute care setting, it is important to identify all healthcare workers who have contact of any kind or duration with patients in your microsystem.

Long-term care residents, because of the nature of their setting, have the ability to get to know the professionals who work within their microsystem quite well. Nursing assistants are a crucial part of the care delivery system, providing the majority of daily care for the residents. Certainly, nurses oversee the care of each patient; however, in many instances, the nursing assistants actually deliver the care. Also, the housekeeping and dietary professionals play a more significant role in long-term care, delivering services that patients can no longer provide for themselves. The provider role in long-term care usually consists of Medicare or Medicaid-determined visit frequency, all the while relying on nursing staff to notify the provider if resident condition or needs change. Activity opportunities, spiritual services, and transportation services are often provided within the facility. Ancillary services such as laboratory, radiology, pharmacy, and rehabilitation are frequently contracted from other facilities, although some long-term care facilities provide these services in-house. As this is the resident's home, a core group of professionals contributing to care is common, and residents rely on them to bring in other professionals as needed.

Processes

Microsystem experts Nelson, Batalden, and Godfrey (2007) suggest "beginning to have all staff understand the processes of care and services in your practice is a key to developing a common understanding and focus for improvement" (p. 408). In all healthcare settings, a common process to be analyzed includes safe movement of the patient through the individual microsystem and even further through the healthcare continuum (Exhibit 4.4). Questions to ask in all settings may include, "What does entry into this setting require?" "How do we assist patients through the new patient process?" "What

Exhibit 4.4

The Processes Portion of the Inpatient Unit Profile 5P Assessment Template

D. Know Your Processes: How do things get done in the microsystem? Who does what? What are the step-by-step processes? How long does the care process take? Where are the delays? What are the "between" microsystems hand-offs?

1. Create Flow Charts of Routine Processes.	Do You Use/Initiate Any of the Following?	Capacity	# Rooms _____	# Beds _____
	Check all that apply		# Turnovers/Bed/Year _____	

a) Overall admission and treatment process
b) Admit to Inpatient Unit
c) Usual Inpatient Care
d) Change of Shift Process
e) Discharge Process
f) Transfer to Another Facility process
g) Medication Administration
h) Adverse Event

☐ Standing Orders/Critical Pathways
☐ Rapid Response Team
☐ Bed Management Rounds
☐ Multidisciplinary/with Family Rounds
☐ Midnight Rounds
☐ Preceptor/Charge Role
☐ Discharge Goals

Linking Microsystems
(e.g., ED, ICU, Skilled Nursing Facility)

2. *Complete the Core and Supporting Process Assessment Tool, p. 14.*

Source: The Dartmouth Institute Microsystem Academy, Godfrey, M., Nelson, E., & Batalden, P.; Institute of Medicine. (2005). *Microsystem Academy Knowledge Center: Inpatient Workbook* (p. 6). Retrieved from http://clinicalmicrosystem.org/knowledge-center/workbooks/.

processes do we have in place to maintain patient privacy, safety, and comfort?" "How is care delivered in this microsystem?" "Does this patient require well care or sick care?" and, finally, "What risks could the patient encounter by being present within this microsystem?" (Nelson, Batalden, & Godfrey, 2007). Answering these questions and creating a visual representation of the workflow, such as a process map, will help you and other professionals in your microsystem understand the need for process improvement (Nelson, Batalden, & Godfrey, 2007).

Essential Facts

Process mapping is a method for creating a diagram that uses graphic symbols to show the steps and the flow of a process. Other commonly used names for a process map are flow diagram and flowchart (Nelson, Batalden, & Godfrey, 2007, p. 298).

As primary care is generally where patients enter the healthcare system, it makes sense to examine a patient's initial interaction with the healthcare system and their future plan of care. Many patients are proactive with their medical care, requesting preventive screenings and well care, whereas others plan to visit the primary care provider for chronic disease management or illness only. Identifying patients' plans of action is key when analyzing processes within primary care. Within acute care and ambulatory settings, the multitude of processes that exist focus upon planned versus emergency care and, therefore, well or ill entry into the microsystem. Those patients having babies or elective surgeries may not be without illness but currently are in an acceptable state of health, allowing them to proceed with a preexisting plan. Looking at processes that are directly related to care of the well patient is important here, such as preadmission testing, early registration, and assessment of discharge needs. Conversely, those patients entering a hospital or utilizing urgent care on an emergency or unplanned basis will likely be more concerned regarding the timeline for treatment. "How long will I be in the hospital?" is many times the first question asked by those admitted to acute care settings. Examining time-sensitive processes such as test scheduling or in-hospital consultant visits may be productive here. Long-term care processes frequently focus more on quality of life and interaction with family and friends; honing processes in an effort to provide an atmosphere most like the resident's home is the goal.

Patterns

According to Nelson, Batalden, and Godfrey (2007), "patterns exist in every microsystem but often go unnoticed, unacknowledged, or unleveraged" (p. 263). Collecting and analyzing the data of the 5P assessment will reveal microsystem processes in need of quality improvement (Exhibit 4.5). Also, getting staff involved in data collection and analysis encourages them to recognize current and future process issues and bring them to you, the CNL, to implement resolution strategies. Frontline staff are in a perfect position to discover deficiencies within their microsystem and, many times, have great ideas on how to solve the process issues they find.

After the 5P assessment is complete, the final step in microsystem assessment is to determine what metrics are important for quality improvement within your unit. What are the metrics that matter (MTM) within your microsystem? To determine these, CNLs must answer the what, why, and how questions related to performance (Nelson, Batalden, & Godfrey, 2007). Questions to ask include "What are the most important performance measures your microsystem recognizes?" "Why are these metrics important?" and "How might you use these metrics to improve the quality of care within your

Exhibit 4.5

The Patterns Portion of the Inpatient Unit Profile 5P Assessment Template

E. Know Your Patterns: What patterns are present but not acknowledged in your microsystem? What is the leadership and social pattern? How often does the microsystem meet to discuss patient care? Are patients and families involved? What are your results and outcomes?

- Does every member of the unit meet regularly as a team?
- How frequently?

- Do the members of the unit regularly review and discuss safety and reliability issues?

- What have you successfully changed?
- What are you most proud of?
- What is your financial picture?

- What is the most significant pattern of variation?

Complete "Metrics that Matter," pp. 20 and 21.

Source: The Dartmouth Institute Microsystem Academy, Godfrey, M., Nelson, E., & Batalden, P.; Institute of Medicine. (2005). *Microsystem Academy Knowledge Center: Inpatient Workbook* (p. 6). Retrieved from http://clinicalmicrosystem.org/knowledge-center/workbooks/.

microsystem?" (Nelson, Batalden, & Godfrey, 2007). For assistance, the *Microsystem Academy Knowledge Center* has resources such as the *Metrics Than Matter* portion of the workbooks as well as the *Measure What Matters* worksheet.

THE NEXT STEP

Essential Facts

The purpose of assessing is to make an informed and correct overall diagnosis of your microsystem. First, identify and celebrate the strengths of your system. Second, identify and consider opportunities to improve your system (Nelson, Batalden, & Godfrey, 2007, p. 421).

Nelson, Batalden, and Godfrey (2007) posit "assessing the 5 Ps and then reflecting on their connections and interdependence often reveals new improvement and redesign opportunities" (p. 389). Putting all of the pieces together (Exhibit 4.6) is your first step postassessment.

The State of the Microsystem

Not unlike the State of the Union address that occurs every January in the United States, the state of the microsystem meeting determines what the current needs are and prepares us for the work to be done in coming months. According to Nelson, Batalden, and Godfrey (2007), a five-step workshop-style meeting can be an appropriate method to do just this, with a suggested format as follows:

1. Assign a meeting leader, facilitator, timekeeper, and recorder prior to starting. Develop an agenda and timeline to cover all five steps in this exercise. Be sure to assign enough time for the team to cover each of the exercise steps. Plan enough time at the end of all the sessions to synthesize the information and prepare a report.
2. Prepare five envelopes that contain preliminary information from your microsystem about the 5Ps (purpose, patients, professionals, processes, patterns), one P per envelope. Some important information will be available, and some will not. Use the workbook to help you identify the data needed to assess and diagnose your microsystem. Focus on one P at a time. It is important to review

Exhibit 4.6

The Complete Inpatient Unit Profile 5P Assessment Template

Inpatient Unit Profile

A. Purpose:
Why does your unit exist?

Administrative Director:　　　　Site Contact:　　　　Date:

　　　　　　　　　　　　　　　　Nurse Director:　　　　Medical Director:

B. Know Your Patients: Take a close look into your unit, create a "high-level" picture of the patient population that you serve. Who are they? What resources do they use? How do the patients view the care they receive?

Est. Age Distribution of Pts.:	%	List Your Top 10 Diagnoses/ Conditions		Pt. Satisfaction Scores	% Always
19–50 years		1.	6.	Nurses	
51–65 years		2.	7.	Doctors	
66–75 years		3.	8.	Environment	
76+ years		4	9.	Pain	
		5.	10.	Discharge	% Yes
% Females				Overall	% Excellent

(continued)

Exhibit 4.6

The Complete Inpatient Unit Profile 5P Assessment Template (continued)

Living Situation	%	Point of Entry	%	Pt. Population Census: Do These Numbers Change by Season? (Y/N)	Y/N
Married		Admissions		Pt. Census by Hour	
Domestic Partner		Clinic		Pt. Census by Day	
Live Alone		ED		Pt. Census by Week	
Live With Others		Transfer		Pt. Census by Year	
Skilled Nursing Facility		**Discharge Disposition**	**%**	30-Day Readmit Rate	
Nursing Home		Home		Our Pats. in Other Units	
Homeless		Home With Visiting Nurse		Off Service Pts. on Our Unit	
Patient Type	**LOS avg. Range**	Skilled Nursing Facility		Frequency of Inability to Admit Pts.	
Medical		Other Hospital		***Complete "Through the Eyes of Your Patient", p. 8.***	
Surgical		Rehab Facility			
Mortality Rate		Transfer to ICU			

C. Know Your Professionals: Use the following template to create a comprehensive picture of your unit. Who does what and when? Is the right person doing the right activity? Are roles being optimized? Are all roles who contribute to the patient experience listed?

Current Staff	Day FTEs	Evening FTEs	Night FTEs	Weekend FTEs	Overtime by Role	Admitting Medical Service	%
MD Total						Internal Medicine	
Hospitalists Total						Hematology/Oncology	
Unit Leader Total						Pulmonary	
CNSs Total						Family Practice	
RNs Total						ICU	
LPNs Total						Other	
LNAs Total						**Supporting Diagnostic Departments**	
Residents Total							
Technicians Total						(e.g., Respiratory, Lab, Cardiology, Pulmonary, Radiology)	
Secretaries Total							
Clinical Resource Coord.							
Social Worker							
Health Service Assts.							
Ancillary Staff							

(continued)

Exhibit 4.6

The Complete Inpatient Unit Profile 5P Assessment Template (*continued*)

			Staff Satisfaction Scores	
Do you Use Per Diems?	____ Yes	____ No	How stressful is the unit?	____ % Not Satisfied
Do You Use Travelers?	____ Yes	____ No	Would you recommend it as a good place to work?	____ % Strongly Agree
Do You Use On-Call Staff?	____ Yes	____ No		
Do You Use a Float Pool?	____ Yes	____ No		

*Each staff member should complete the Personal Skills Assessment and "The Activity Survey," pp. 10–12.

D. Know Your Processes: How do things get done in the microsystem? Who does what? What are the step-by-step processes? How long does the care process take? Where are the delays? What are the "between" microsystems hand-offs?

2. Create Flow Charts of Routine Processes.

a) Overall admission and treatment process
b) Admit to Inpatient Unit
c) Usual Inpatient Care
d) Change of Shift Process
e) Discharge Process

Do You Use/Initiate Any of the Following? Check all that apply

- ☐ Standing Orders/Critical Pathways _____
- ☐ Rapid Response Team
- ☐ Bed Management Rounds
- ☐ Multidisciplinary/With Family Rounds

Capacity # Turnovers/Bed/Year _____

Linking Microsystems

(e.g., ED, ICU, Skilled Nursing Facility)

Rooms _____   # Beds _____

f) Transfer to Another Facility Process ☐ Midnight Rounds

g) Medication Administration ☐ Preceptor/Charge Role

h) Adverse Event ☐ Discharge Goals

2. *Complete the Core and Supporting Process Assessment Tool, p. 14.*

E. Know Your Patterns: What patterns are present but not acknowledged in your microsystem? What is the leadership and social pattern? How often does the microsystem meet to discuss patient care? Are patients and families involved? What are your results and outcomes?

- Does every member of the unit meet regularly as a team?
- How frequently?
- What is the most significant pattern of variation?

- Do the members of the unit regularly review and discuss safety and reliability issues?

- What have you successfully changed?
- What are you most proud of?
- What is your financial picture?

*Complete "Metrics that Matter," pp. 20 and 21.

Source: The Dartmouth Institute Microsystem Academy; Godfrey, M. Nelson, E., & Batalden, P.; Institute of Medicine. (2005). *Microsystem Academy Knowledge Center: Inpatient Workbook* (p. 6). Retrieved from http://clinicalmicrosystem.org/knowledge-center/workbooks/.

the data, determine what additional information is needed and where it may be obtained, and then move to the next P.
3. Use the microsystem workbook to determine which tools will help the lead improvement team to gain deeper insight into the microsystem. Some of the needed microsystem information is in each of the envelopes that you prepared; the microsystem workbook can help you to assess and diagnose your microsystem, and it provides additional tools for collecting desired information.
4. When reviewing each P, some of the questions that follow this exercise may facilitate the team discussion.
5. At the end of the 5Ps series, the lead improvement team will have a deeper awareness of its microsystem and can report back to all the microsystem members and summarize the learning and conclusions. The lead improvement team will also know what additional information it needs to deepen its own knowledge about its microsystem (p. 264).

Questions to discuss within the group might include "Do the mission statements of both the organization and microsystem align? If not, how could we update the microsystem mission statement?" "What do you notice after evaluating the data collection regarding patients, professionals, processes, and patterns? Do you need additional information? If so, where might you secure this information?" and "Are there any conclusions you can draw from these data? How could the microsystem workbook help?" (Nelson, Batalden, & Godfrey, 2007). Finally, create a pictorial report in the form of a 5Ps wall model (found at the Microsystem Academy Knowledge Center), and post in a highly visible place for all microsystem members to see and discuss.

> ### Clinical Nurse Leader Vignette 4.1:
> ### Assessing Your Microsystem: Reducing Pressure Ulcers in an ICU Unit
>
> "What? Our pressure ulcer rate is up? Well, we do have pretty sick people here you know." Our ICU unit goal was to take great care of critically ill patients and not introduce them to new sources of harm. After all, they were sick enough when they came to the ICU in the first place! But what had changed?
>
> Patient type was consistent, with respiratory failure, critical trauma, cardiac and neurosurgical and sepsis being our primary diagnoses. On both shifts, ICU professionals consisted of nurses,

nursing assistants, secretaries, physicians, pharmacists, respiratory therapists, and many ancillary staff. There were differences between the shifts, with nursing assistants only working at night and secretaries, dieticians, wound care nurses, and physical therapists working only during the day.

Countless processes were in place to maintain unit function and reduce risk of pressure ulcers in ICU patients. We turned patients every 2 hours, assessed skin every 4 hours, charted a Braden scale every 12 hours, and kept patients' skin dry: Where was the gap in this pressure ulcer prevention process that was allowing skin breakdown? After evaluating ICU pressure ulcer rates and types, the statistics showed a pattern of occurrence in those patients with life sustaining respiratory devices, such as endotracheal tubes, bipap masks, and nasal cannulas. Pressure ulcers in common places such as heels, elbows, and coccyx were not occurring; all pressure ulcers were respiratory device related.

This was good and bad all at the same time! The ICU staff was doing a great job following skin care polices, as reflected in the lack of pressure ulcers in usual areas, yet, we had pressure ulcers occurring around life sustaining devices we couldn't remove. Had anything truly changed in the care staff delivered? Or were we simply finally connecting the dots within our microsystem with a CNL guiding the pen? After forming a transdisciplinary committee and evaluating the data, a detailed quality improvement plan was implemented, which resulted in zero-pressure ulcers for the subsequent 12 months.

Ann Deerhake, DNP, RN, CNL, CCRN

References

American Academy of Family Physicians. (2019). *Primary care*. Retrieved from https://www.aafp.org/about/policies/all/primary-care.html

American Society of Healthcare Engineering. (2017). *Eight ambulatory models of care*. Retrieved from https://www.hfmmagazine.com/articles/1852-eight-ambulatory-models-of-care

The Dartmouth Institute Microsystem Academy, Godfrey, M., Nelson, E., Batalden, P., & Institute of Medicine. (2005). *Microsystem Academy Knowledge Center: Inpatient Workbook*. Retrieved from http://clinicalmicrosystem.org/knowledge-center/workbooks/

L'Ecuyer, K., Shatto, B., Hoffmann, R., & Crecelius, M. (2016). The certified clinical nurse leader in critical care. *Dimensions of Critical Care Nursing: DCCN, 35*(5), 248–254. doi:10.1097/DCC.0000000000000202

McKeon, L., Norris, T., Webb, S., Hix, C., Ramsey, G., & Jacob, S. (2009). Teaching clinical nurse leaders how to diagnose the clinical microsystem. *Journal of Professional Nursing, 25*(6), 373–378. doi:10.1016/j.profnurs.2009.04.001

National Academy of Sciences. (1999). *To err is human: Building a safer healthcare system.* Retrieved from http://www.nationalacademies.org/hmd/~/media/Files/Report%20Files/1999/To-Err-is-Human/To%20Err%20is%20Human%201999%20%20report%20brief.pdf

Nelson, E., Batalden, P., & Godfrey, M. (2007). *Quality by design: A clinical microsystems approach.* San Francisco, CA: Jossey-Bass.

Rankin, V., Ralyea, T., & Sotomayor, G. (2018). Clinical nurse leaders forging the path of population health. *Journal of Professional Nursing, 34*(4), 269–272. doi:10.1016/j.profnurs.2017.10.008

Rickles, D., Hawe, P., & Shiell, A. (2007). A simple guide to chaos and complexity. *Journal of Epidemiology and Community, 61*(11), 933–937. doi:10.1136/jech.2006.054254

Rodziewicz, T., & Hipskind, J. (2019). *Medical error prevention.* Treasure Island FL: StatPearls Publishing. Retrieved from https://www.ncbi.nlm.nih.gov/books/NBK499956/

Schein, E. (2017). *Organizational culture and leadership* [Kindle ed.]. The Jossey-Bass Business & Management Series. Hoboken, NJ: Wiley.

Wilson, L., Orff, S., Gerry, T., Shirley, B. R., Tabor, D., Caiazzo, K., & Rouleau, D. (2013). Evolution of an innovative role: The clinical nurse leader. *Journal of Nursing Management, 21*(1), 175–181. doi:10.1111/j.1365-2834.2012.01454.x

5

Utilizing Evidence to Improve Practice

Janice Wilcox

"Take nothing on its looks; take everything on evidence. There's no better rule."

~Charles Dickens

INTRODUCTION

The American Association of Colleges of Nursing (AACN, 2007) states that the clinical nurse leader (CNL) "designs, implements, and evaluates care by coordinating, delegating and supervising the care provided by the health care team" (p. 6). The educational and practice competencies for the CNL outline the knowledge and expertise the CNL should hold in order to be able to coordinate care and supervise teams. The third AACN (2013) CNL assumption states that "practice guidelines are based on evidence" (p. 7). Therefore, understanding how to incorporate evidence into practice and lead the utilization of evidence by the healthcare team is an essential component of CNL practice.

After reading this chapter, you will be able to:

1. Describe the relevance of evidence to nursing practice and patient outcomes
2. Classify literature according to type of evidence
3. Analyze statistical significance of evidence
4. Recognize common search strategies
5. Identify barriers of incorporation of evidence-based practice (EBP) within systems
6. Identify potential interventions to instill team value of EBP.

HISTORICAL PERSPECTIVE OF EBP

The pivotal Institute of Medicine's (IOM) *Crossing the Quality Chasm* (2001) report brought to light the need for consistent practice based on evidence. Even though the Cochrane database, which houses systematic reviews of current research, was initiated in the 1970s, physicians were continuing to practice based on their own beliefs and teachings (Mackey & Bassendowski, 2017). This was also true of nurses. Many of the procedures and skills that nurses performed were based on what was taught in their formal educational programs or organizational traditions, and not from current evidence. The IOM (2001) report discussed how practice should be based on evidence obtained from research and not passed on from clinician to clinician. The report also highlighted the fact that there was a lengthy period of time from when research findings were disseminated and when they were actually integrated into the practice setting. The IOM felt this gap should be closed to allow quicker application of research within clinical settings (IOM, 2001).

According to Mackey and Bassendowski (2017), nursing's history of EBP dates back to Florence Nightingale. Nightingale performed research on environmental factors affecting patient outcomes and changed practice according to her findings. One example of her work corresponds to current changes in patient care in many organizations. She compared the utilization of different bathing principles, cold water, hot water, and soap, to determine which had the greatest benefit in increasing cleanliness; her findings determined hot water and soap resulted in the best outcomes (Mackey & Bassendowski, 2017). Today, many organizations have replaced bathing with soap and water to bathing with chlorhexidine wipes as a means of preventing hospital-acquired infections (Denny & Munro, 2017; Patel et al., 2019). Nightingale's quest to refine practice that elicits the best possible patient outcomes was the precursor to successors' work in improving patient care.

Essential Facts

"In a little book on nursing, published a short time ago, we are told, that, 'with proper care it is very seldom that the windows cannot be opened for a few minutes twice in the day to admit fresh air from without.' I should think not; nor twice in the hour either. It only shows how little the subject has been considered" (Nightingale, 1860, p. 9).

RELEVANCE TO PRACTICE

Many organizations and disciplines have defined EBP. David Sackett and colleagues worked diligently in driving the EBP movement in medicine. Their definition states that evidence-based medicine is "the conscientious, explicit, and judicious use of current best evidence in making decisions about the care of individual patients" (Sackett, Rosenberg, Gray, Haynes, & Richardson, 1996, p. 71). Melnyk, Fineout-Overholt, Stillwell, and Williamson (2010) distinguish evidence-based nursing practice as "a problem solving approach to the delivery of healthcare that integrates the best evidence from well-designed studies and patient care data, and combines it with patient preferences and values and nurse expertise" (p. 51). Morin (2010) acknowledges that "irrespective of the definition employed, key elements of evidence-based practice include addressing a clinical problem or question by examining the best available scientific evidence and then integrating that evidence with patient preferences and practitioner expertise" (p. 1).

Simply put, EBP is the utilization of the best evidence to answer clinical questions on the most beneficial treatments, processes, procedures, and actions used by nurses in the care of their patients. Along with utilizing evidence, however, the nurse must also consider the patient's preferences in the provision of care while bringing in their own expertise. The patient preference aspect is extremely important as treatments must coincide with the patient's beliefs, culture, and experiences in order for the treatment to be followed and be beneficial to the patient. This corresponds well with the recent call for patient-centered care. The nurse's clinical expertise involves the ability of the nurse to utilize current knowledge in appropriately and effectively performing skills in a timely manner, identifying and managing benefits and risks resulting from the skill, and the ability to transfer knowledge and skills to similar patient situations (Sigma Theta Tau, 2008).

Basing practice on evidence has many benefits to organizations and patients. Today's healthcare systems are attempting to manage costs due to Medicare and insurance provider value-based payment models while maintaining high reliability practices. Organizations are struggling to improve outcomes, decrease lengths of stay, reduce rehospitalizations, and manage hospital-acquired injuries. Standardized EBPs can assist with these struggles as they "reduce inconsistencies in care and improve quality and patient safety while also containing costs" (Warren et al., 2016, p. 15). Using current knowledge also permits organizations to make better predictions regarding outcomes when EBP practices are initiated, along with enhancing the analysis process to determine potential gaps (Stevens, 2013). The greatest benefit of utilizing EBP, however, is ensuring patients are receiving the best possible care, leading to the best possible patient outcomes.

Essential Facts

CNLs can role model Melnyk et al.'s "Step 0: Cultivate a Spirit of Inquiry" within the entire microsystem by starting with these questions:

Who can I seek out to assist me in enhancing my evidence-based practice (EBP) knowledge and skills and serve as my EBP mentor?

Which of my practices are currently evidence based, and which don't have any evidence to support them?

When is the best time to question my current clinical practices, and with whom?

Where can I find the best evidence to answer my clinical questions?

Why am I doing what I do with my patients?

How can I become more skilled in EBP and mentor others to implement evidence-based care? (Melnyk et al., 2009, p. 51)

STEPS IN THE EBP PROCESS

The PICOT Question

The EBP process consists of steps to move from asking questions to dissemination of findings. This usually begins with asking a clinical question utilizing a PICOT question format. The letters in PICOT correspond with Problem/patient, Intervention of interest, Comparison of another intervention, the Outcome of interest, and Timeframe (Stillwell, Fineout-Overhold, Melynk, & Williamson, 2010a, p. 59). The PICOT question format permits key terms to be easily identified and inserted into library database search engines.

An example may be as follows: In (P) congestive heart failure patients, how does the use of (I) printed educational materials (C) compare with the use of online video educational materials affect the (O) patient's knowledge level and ability to provide self-care (T) prior to discharge?

Searching for Evidence

A next step is searching for the evidence. If your organization provides access to a library, you can use different databases within the library to search for current research. Common databases include the Cochrane Database of Systematic Reviews, PubMed, EBSCO, and CINAHL. If you do not have access to a library, you can search the Cochrane Database by going through their website at www.cochrane.org. PubMed can also be accessed without a library database at https://www.ncbi.nlm.nih.gov/pubmed. Your organization could also connect to databases through the Joanna Briggs Institute at https://www.joannabriggs.org. This site offers access to current studies and information on EBP. Clinical guidelines may also be used to guide practice, and these can be found at https://guidelines.ecri.org. Prior to accessing guidelines, the user must set up a free account. See Table 5.1 for listing of databases and websites.

Utilizing search strategies such as using keywords and phrases along with Boolean operators, such as *and, or,* and *not,* combine words and phrases to increase the likelihood of obtaining the most relevant literature. Limiting the variables within the search is possible by selecting certain categories within the database such as narrowing

Table 5.1

Common Databases for Current Healthcare Research	
Cochrane Database of Systematic Reviews	www.cochrane.org
PubMed	https://www.ncbi.nlm.nih.gov/pubmed
Joanna Briggs Institute	https://www.joannabriggs.org
Clinical Guidelines	http://guidelines.ecri.org

the dates of publication, types of publications, journal subsets, types of research, or other available choices.

When searching for literature, it is best to have an idea of what the best evidence may be for your particular project. There are different categories of quantitative research studies, and the category will determine the strength of the research and findings. This is often referred to as the level of evidence. The level of evidence is important as higher level evidence provides clinicians with greater confidence that the interventions performed within the research are worthwhile (Stillwell et al., 2010b). Systematic reviews and meta-analyses are considered the highest level with randomized controlled trials and cohort studies being second and third on the list. Cross-sectional surveys, case studies, and qualitative research are the fourth-level evidence, and expert opinion is considered the lowest-level evidence.

As a review, systematic reviews and meta-analyses synthesize and analyze evidence from randomized controlled trials. Randomized control trials are experiments where the subjects are randomly selected to an experimental or control group. Controlled trials without randomization are experiments that involve subjects who are not randomly assigned to a treatment or control group. Case-controlled studies are studies that compare subjects with a certain condition or illness with another group who do not have the condition or illness. A cohort study involves observing a certain group at various points in time (Stillwell et al., 2010b). Qualitative studies can be beneficial to the potential project or organizational initiative as well, but fall below the expert opinion level on the hierarchy since qualitative studies do not measure statistical significance. When compiling literature for a project, it is best then to have several higher level research articles that provide the best evidence that you should continue with the noted intervention.

Critical Appraisal of the Evidence

Essential Facts

Rapid critical appraisal of evidence starts with determining if study results are valid, vital, and valuable to patient care (Melnyk et al., 2010).

Critical appraisal requires nurses to have an idea of how validity and reliability are determined. When selecting articles, you are attempting to find literature that is relevant and applicable to your project and have valid and reliable research results. Determining validity and reliability may be difficult for nurses who are not familiar with statistical measures of research. Some organizations have nurse scientists who can assist in interpreting statistical outcomes. There are also many texts and websites that offer insight into interpretation of research results. Typically, when appraising evidence, you will examine the statistical significance or p value. The p value is a probability range, and most studies use a threshold of .05 for a p value. A .05 p value means that there is less than a 5% chance the results of the study occurred by accident.

A study may also describe an odds ratio (OR), which is a relative measure of effect. This permits comparison of the intervention group with the control group. When calculating the ratio, the intervention group is the numerator, and the control group is the denominator. If the calculation result is one, it implies that there is no difference between the intervention and the control group. If the OR is greater than 1, it indicates that the control is better than the intervention. If the OR is less than 1, the intervention is better than the control.

Confidence intervals (CIs) can also be examined. CIs describe the range of an effect within a certain degree of certainty. A 95% CI is the range where one can be 95% confident that the actual values or results fall within the upper and lower limits of a range. For example, if a trial is comparing a certain drug to a placebo, the authors may use the OR and CI, stating OR 0.5 95% CI 0.4–0.6. This would indicate that the odds of a death in the intervention group is 50% less than that in the placebo group with the true population effect between 60% and 40%.

Another criterion to examine is the sample of experimental studies. How large is the sample and how many participants withdrew during the study? Was there discussion of why participants withdrew? Finally, you need to determine if the study participants and environment are similar to your own patients and unit. Will the intervention and results transfer to your population of patients? You should be able to gain insight from reading the discussion section of the article. This section should answer the research question, provide meaning to the results, provide information on weaknesses or limitations of the study, and include recommendations for future studies. Once you determine the study strength, you will be able to decide if it is worth incorporating into your EBP project.

Implementing EBP Change

Now that you have compiled a collection of relevant evidence, it is time to determine if a practice change should be made. Be sure that the intervention will transfer to your population and coincide with clinical expertise and organizational culture. Consulting with other nurses, managers, and administrators is beneficial to determine feasibility of a practice change. You will also need to obtain buy-in from stakeholders, especially if the project will incur additional costs. Development of an action plan that includes things such as project time frame, costs, educational support and programs, supplies, and potential barriers will be necessary in moving forward with an initiative. It is often best to pilot or trial the change on one unit or with one particular population of patients. EBP changes are often introduced as quality improvement (QI) initiatives utilizing QI tools and principles. You will need to think about the process of change and apply change theories and philosophies as any new practice change will be met with some resistance. Be sure to identify the innovators and early adopters to assist in gaining buy-in from staff.

Evaluate Outcomes and Dissemination

Following the implementation of the change, evaluation of the impact on the outcome of interest is performed. Evaluation should be performed throughout the change process to address any barriers or concerns that are identified. Again, QI tools can be used for evaluation purposes. Quality metrics such as nurse-sensitive indicators may be useful if the intervention focuses on one of these areas. Besides evaluating system or patient outcomes, you should also be evaluating process measures. Determine if there are any processes that interfere with the EBP intervention that can be affecting the patient or system outcome. Process measures may involve looking at the supply chain to determine if supplies are available when staff require them or if delays are occurring in procedures due to patient movement from area to area. If the change is not eliciting the desired effect, it may be that a process needs updating rather than an entirely new intervention. Whether the outcomes are beneficial or not, it is important to disseminate the findings to others within the organization and through other means such as publication and conferences. Dissemination will assist others in determining if the particular EBP change could be beneficial to their setting or if they should consider other options.

MODELS AND RESOURCES

Essential Facts

Selecting and applying a model for evidence-based practice change provides a framework to guide the CNL during introduction and implementation of change within the microsystem.

There are different models and resources that can assist in moving through the EBP process. Each model goes through the basic steps of asking clinical questions, searching for evidence, appraising evidence, translating evidence into practice, and dissemination of findings. However, each model goes through the steps slightly differently; therefore, depending upon the organizational needs and philosophies, one model may be preferred over another. The Virginia Office of Nursing Service created a table comparing four different process steps; the link can be found in Table 5.2.

The John Hopkins Evidence-Based Practice Model consists of three criteria: practice question, evidence, and translation. Within each criterion are steps that permit the user to complete the process of asking the clinical question, searching and appraising the evidence, and translating the evidence into practice (Newhouse, Dearholt, Poe, Pugh, & White, 2007). The Johns Hopkins Center for Evidence-Based Practice website grants permission to utilize templates that guide each step of the process. After being granted permission, the templates can be printed or electronically downloaded for ease of use. See Appendix 5.1.

Melnyk et al. (2010) developed a seven-step process, which is similar to the steps in The Johns Hopkins Model; however, they begin with "cultivating a spirit of inquiry" (p. 51) within the system. This refers to engaging nurses in critically looking at their practice and providing encouragement in utilizing critical thinking by questioning the procedures and processes utilized in caring for their patients. These authors have written a series of articles that are available online through the *American Journal of Nursing;* these articles provide examples of moving through the EBP process.

The Iowa Model begins with identifying "triggering issues and opportunities" (Iowa Model Collaborative, 2017, p. 1) that are

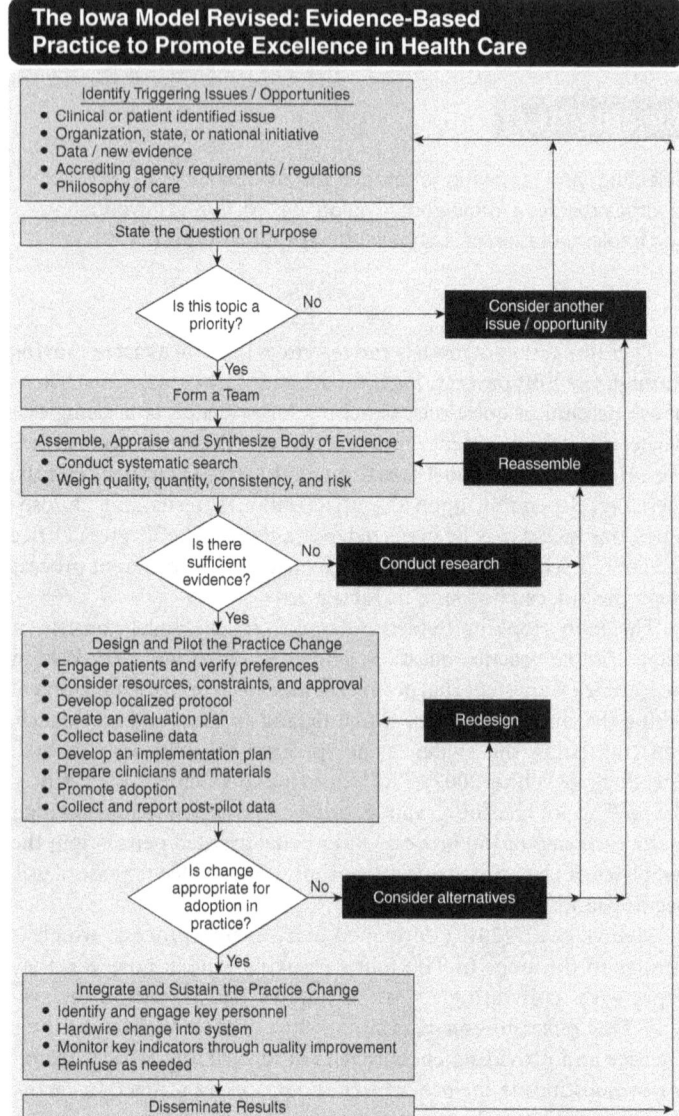

Figure 5.1 The Iowa Model of evidence-based practice to promote quality care.

Source: Reprinted with permission from the University of Iowa Hospitals and Clinics, Copyright 2015.

significant priorities to patient care and the organization. A major difference in this model is that it emphasizes the importance of the entire organization and individuals within the organization in moving practice decisions forward (Figure 5.1). This is exemplified in the second step, which is slightly different than other models, as it requires a team to be formed to handle the activities of the EBP process. The team includes major stakeholders related to the "trigger," and each member has a role in the entire process. Following the formation of the team, the process of searching and appraising evidence begins.

The Stevens Star Model of Knowledge Transformation uses a five-point star to illustrate the five concepts or elements of knowledge in sequential form that are necessary to integrate knowledge into practice (Figure 5.2). Parkosewich (2013) states that a major difference between this model and others is that "it provides more conceptual discussions about each of the stages opposed to prescribing tangible steps to use within each stage ... and allows for orderly progression of knowledge across [the] five conceptual domains" (p. 73). The domains consist of discovery research, evidence summary, translation guidelines, practice integration and process, and outcome evaluation. Further information on this model can be found at the University of Texas School of Nursing site found in Table 5.2.

McMaster's University developed a model called evidence-informed decision-making. This is a five-step model that integrates the concepts of clinical expertise, aspects of the clinical setting, patient preferences, research, and healthcare resources. The website

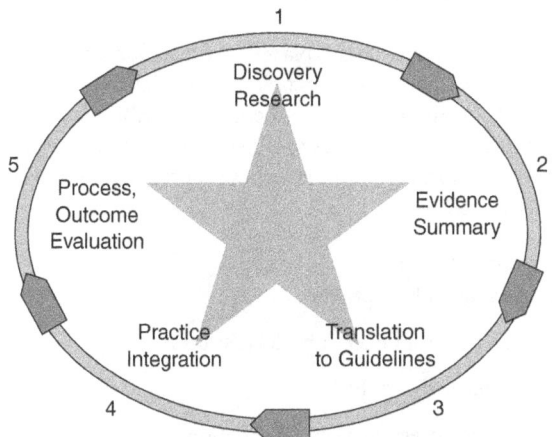

Figure 5.2 Stevens Star Model of Knowledge Transformation.

Source: Reprinted with permission. Copyright Stevens 2015. Stevens Star Model of Knowledge Transformation.

Table 5.2

Evidence-Based Practice Models

Model	Weblink
The John Hopkins Evidence-Based Practice Model	https://www.hopkinsmedicine.org/evidence-based-practice/ijhn_2017_ebp.html
Melynk & Fineout-Overholt EBP Process *American Journal of Nursing* Series	https://www.nursingcenter.com/evidencebasedpracticenetwork/home/tools-resources/collections/ajn-ebp-series.aspx
University of Iowa Model	www.uiowacsomaygeroresources.com/category-s/149.htm
Star Model of Knowledge Transformation	http://nursing.aahs.org/wp-content/uploads/The-ACE-Star-Model.pdf http://nursing.uthscsa.edu/onrs/starmodel/star-model.asp
McMaster University Nursing Resources	https://hslmcmaster.libguides.com/friendly.php?s=nursing
Virginia Office of Nursing Services Comparison of EBP Process Steps	https://www.va.gov/nursing/ebp/docs/EBP_ProcessComparisonStepsCurriculumHandout_www.pdf

(see Table 5.2) provides many resources such as PICOT template, search strategies, and appraisal tools.

MANAGING BARRIERS TO EBP

Even though great emphasis is placed on the importance and benefits of EBP practice, not all organizations, clinicians, and nurses have embraced it. Common barriers to embracing EBP have been noted in recent studies on the status of EBP within organizations nationally and globally. From these studies, common barriers were noted and consist of the following:

1. Perceived lack of time
2. Lack of value in EBP practice

   a. Resistance from peers/physicians/nurse leaders

3. Lack of knowledge of EBP

   a. Ability to access current information
   b. Search strategies skills
   c. Ability to appraise evidence

4. Lack of resources to search for evidence

   a. Available resources

5. Organizational culture
6. Lack of authority/power to initiate EBP changes (Duncomb, 2018; Melnyk & Fineout-Overholt, 2012; Melnyk, Gallagher-Ford, Long, & Fineout-Overholt, 2014; Parkosewich, 2013; Sadoughi, Azadi, & Azadi, 2017; Warren et al., 2016)

These studies also determined that the educational and experience levels of nurses were factors in appreciating the value of EBP. It was noted that nurses with higher levels of education, particularly educated at the master's level, and nurses with fewer years of experience were more likely to engage in EBP practice. It was also shown that Magnet-designated hospitals were more likely to have engaged nurses and consistent EBPs due to the additional resources that these hospitals often have.

As leaders within the clinical setting, it is important for CNLs to recognize and address these barriers. Melnyk and Fineout-Overholt (2012) discuss how mentors have been found to be beneficial in moving past some of these barriers. CNLs, acting as EBP mentors, can assist nurses in instilling a sense of inquiry and innovation within the nursing team as well as guiding nurses through the EBP process. CNLs can educate nurses on how to access databases, create PICOT questions, search for evidence, and how to move an initiative forward. A CNL can begin by emulating characteristics that enhance a culture embracing EBP by asking questions about why certain practices are performed and looking for evidence that provides potential improvements in processes.

Journal clubs have been used in clinical nursing for some time to allow for new information to be disseminated. Gardner et al. (2016) initiated a journal club within an intensive care unit and found that nurses were able to apply evidence within the clinical setting. Journal clubs have traditionally been formed to discuss topics or articles but could also be used as a means of teaching nurses how to develop PICOT questions and learn search strategies and how to identify relevant research if computers are available during the meetings. Some organizations have partnered with academic organizations to enlist the assistance of nurse scientists and librarians to act as staff resources.

Many organizations especially those with Magnet status have nursing EBP committees that evaluate practice and potential research interventions. They comprise staff nurses who are seen as clinical leaders within their population of patient and are interested in improving care through EBP. Lack of availability of resources such as computers, databases, and mentors requires CNLs to be advocates for nursing as well as EBP practice by proposing potential benefits to the organization in the way of improving processes and outcomes by the acquisition of these resources. CNLs can be catalysts in changing organizational and microsystem culture, educating nurses, and moving EBP forward while improving outcomes.

Essential Facts

> CNL Competency Essential 4 states that CNLs should work toward the outcome of "facilitat(ing) practice change based on best available evidence that results in quality, safety and fiscally responsible outcomes" (American Association of Colleges of Nursing, 2013, p. 13).

This chapter provides basic principles of EBP. As the EBP movement progresses, more and more educational opportunities are becoming available through in person and online seminars and courses. If assistance in any of the stages of EBP is needed, reach out to academic centers and to the links provided in Table 5.2 to access tools and resources and educational opportunities. As CNLs work to meet the AACN competencies to improve quality and outcomes within the microsystem, lead interdisciplinary teams, and coordinate care, it is essential that engagement in EBP practices occurs. CNLs must also encourage organizations, staff, and interdisciplinary colleagues to embrace these practices as well. Using leadership and change principles along with EBP processes, quality patient outcomes will become a reality, and the worth of the CNL will be acknowledged.

Clinical Nurse Leader Vignette 5.1: Evidence-Based Practice Initiatives in an Acute Cardiac Unit

A communication problem between physicians and nurses was found to be affecting coordination of care and discharge processes within an acute cardiac unit. Andrea, the unit CNL, recalled reading an article on the benefits of physician and nurse rounding and used the Seven Steps of Evidence-Based Practice by Melnyk and

Fineout-Overholt (2015) to determine if this would be a worthwhile option for her unit. She constructed a PICOT question comparing the benefits of physician-only rounding with physician and nurse rounding. Through the literature search and critical appraisal, Andrea found evidence to suggest that physician and nurse rounding enhanced communication by decreasing communication barriers, assisted in eliminating confusion regarding plan of care, and decreased sentinel events by 65%. Buy-in was obtained from a physician group, the nurse manager, and nurse educator on the unit who formed a team to develop the initiative. This team took into consideration the unit values, patient preferences, and clinical expertise of the staff during the development of the project. It was determined to utilize a new call light system, specifically the "MD/NP in room button" to alert nursing staff when physicians were rounding on their patients. The physicians pressed the button, and a notification was sent to the nurse to attend the rounds. The physicians were also provided a daily staffing sheet to indicate the nurse assigned to their patients. Information on the initiative was sent via emails to the nursing staff and specified MD teams to notify them of the intervention and start dates. Education also occurred during staff meetings, and Andrea reinforced the change within the unit on a daily basis. Evaluation of the initiative occurred over a 6-month time period and resulted in enhanced communication among team members, increased patient satisfaction, and increased nurses' satisfaction, as they felt more valued by the physicians. The initiative was then disseminated and then implemented on other units within the organization. Andrea, the CNL, was instrumental in identifying the problem, searching for potential solutions, and overseeing the EBP initiative. Without her insight and skills, the problem may not have been resolved.

References

American Association of Colleges of Nursing. (2013). *Competencies and curricular expectations for clinical nurse leader education and practice.* Retrieved from https://www.aacnnursing.org/Portals/42/AcademicNursing/CurriculumGuidelines/CNL-Competencies-October-2013.pdf

Denny, J., & Munro, C. L. (2017). Chlorhexidine bathing effects on healthcare associated infections. *Biological Research for Nursing, 19*(2), 123–136. doi:10.1177/1099800416654013

Duncomb, D. C. (2018). A multi-institutional study of the perceived barriers and facilitators to implementing evidence-based practice. *Journal of Clinical Nursing, 27*, 1216–1226. doi:10.1111/jocn.14168

Gardner, K., Kanaskie, M. L., Knehans, A. C., Salisbury, S., Doheny, K. K., & Schirm, V. (2016). Implementing and sustaining evidence based practice through a nursing journal club. *Applied Nursing Research, 31*, 139–145. doi:10.1016/j/apnr/2016.02.001

Institute of Medicine. (2001). *Crossing the quality chasm. A new health system for the 21st century.* Washington, DC: The National Academies Press.

Iowa Model Collaborative. (2017). Iowa model of evidence-based practice: Revisions and validation. *Worldviews on Evidence-Based Nursing, 14*(3), 175–182. doi:10.1111/wvn.12223

Mackey, A., & Bassendowski, S. (2017). The history of evidence-based practice in nursing education and practice. *Journal of Professional Nursing, 33*(1), 51–55. doi:10.1016/j.profnurs.2016.05.009

Melnyk, B. M., & Fineout-Overholt, E. (2012). The state of evidence-based practice in U.S. nurses. *The Journal of Nursing Administration, 42*(9), 410–417. doi:10.1097/NNA.0b013e3182664e0a

Melnyk, B. M., & Fineout-Overholt, E. (2015). *Evidence-based practice in nursing & Healthcare. A guide to best practice* (3rd ed.). Philadelphia, PA: Wolters Kluwer Health.

Melnyk, B. M., Fineout-Overholt, E., Stillwell, S. B., & Williamson, K. (2009). Igniting a spirit of inquiry: An essential foundation for evidence-based practice. *American Journal of Nursing, 109*(11), 49–52. doi:10.1097/01.NAJ.0000363354.53883.58

Melnyk, B. M., Fineout-Overholt, E., Stillwell, S. B., & Williamson, K. M. (2010). Evidence-based practice: Step by step: The seven steps of evidence-based practice. *American Journal of Nursing, 110*(1), 51–53. doi:10.1097/01.NAJ.0000366056.06605.d2

Melnyk, B. M., Gallagher-Ford, L., English Long, L., & Fineout-Overholt, E. (2014). The establishment of evidence-based practice competencies for practicing registered nurses and advanced practice nurses in real-world clinical settings: Proficiencies to improve healthcare quality, reliability, patient outcomes, and costs. *Worldviews on Evidence-Based Nursing, 11*(1), 5–15. doi:10.1111/wvn.12021

Morin, K. H. (2010). *Evidence: Critical to practice and education* [Dean's Notes]. Retrieved from https://cna-aiic.ca/-/media/nurseone/page-content/pdf-en/evidence-critical-to-practice-and-education.pdf?la=en&hash=D919334A994E1E2586446DC866229444C6EEE351

Newhouse, R. P., Dearholt, S. L., Poe, S. S., Pugh, L. C., & White, K. M. (2007). *Johns Hopkins nursing evidence-based practice model and guidelines.* Indianapolis, IN: Sigma Theta Tau International.

Nightingale, F. (1860). *Notes on nursing: What it is and what it is not.* New York, NY: D. Appleton and Company.

Parkosewich, J. A. (2013). An infrastructure to advance the scholarly work of staff nurses. *Yale Journal of Biology and Medicine, 86*(1), 63–77.

Patel, A., Parikh, P., Dunn, A. N., Otter, J. A., Thota, P., Fraser, T. G., … Deshpande, A. (2019). Effectiveness of daily chlorhexidine bathing for reducing gram-negative infections: A meta-analysis. *Infection Control & Hospital Epidemiology, 40,* 392–399. doi:10.1017/ice.2019.20

Sackett, D. L., Rosenberg, W. M., Gray, J., Haynes, B., & Richardson, W. S. (1996). Evidence based medicine: What it is and what it isn't. *British Medical Journal, 312*(7023), 71–72. doi:10.1136/bmj.312.7023.71

Sadoughi, F., Azadi, T., & Azadi, T. (2017). Barriers to using electronic evidence based literature in nursing practice: A systematised review. *Health Information and Libraries Journal, 34,* 187–199. doi:10.111/hir.12186

Sigma Theta Tau International 2005–2007 Research and Scholarship Advisory Committee. (2008). Sigma theta tau international position statement on evidence-based practice February 2007 summary. *World Views on Evidence-Based Nursing, 5*(2), 57–59. doi:10.1111/j.1741-6787.2008.00118.x

Stevens, K. (2013, May 31). The impact of evidence-based practice in nursing and the next big ideas. *The Online Journal of Issues in Nursing, 18*(2). doi:10.3912/OJIN.Vol18No02Man04

Stillwell, S. B., Fineout-Overholt, E., Melynk, B. M., & Williamson, K. M. (2010a). Evidence-based practice: Step by step: Asking the clinical question: A key step in evidence-based practice. *American Journal of Nursing, 110*(3), 58–61. doi:10.1097/01.NAJ.0000368959.11129.79

Stillwell, S. B., Fineout-Overholt, E., Melynk, B. M., & Williamson, K. M. (2010b). Evidence-based practice: Step by step: Searching for the evidence. *American Journal of Nursing, 110*(5), 41–47. doi:10.1097/01.NAJ.0000372071.24134.7e

Warren, J. I., McLaughlin, M., Bardsley, J., Eich, J., Esche, C., Kropkowski, L., & Risch, S. (2016). The strengths and challenges of implementing EBP in healthcare systems. *Worldviews on Evidence-Based Nursing, 13*(1), 15–24. doi:10.1111/wvn.12149

Appendix 5.1

JOHNS HOPKINS NURSING EVIDENCE-BASED PRACTICE: PET MANAGEMENT GUIDE

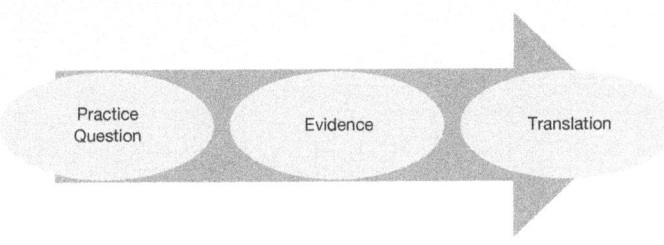

PRACTICE QUESTION

Step 1: Recruit interprofessional team.
Step 2: Define the problem.
Step 3: Develop and refine the EBP question.
Step 4: Identify stakeholders.
Step 5: Determine responsibility for project leadership.
Step 6: Schedule team meetings.

EVIDENCE

Step 7: Conduct internal and external search for evidence.
Step 8: Appraise the level and quality of each piece of evidence.
Step 9: Summarize the individual evidence.
Step 10: Synthesize overall strength and quality of evidence.
Step 11: Develop recommendations for change based on evidence synthesis.

- Strong, compelling evidence, consistent results
- Good evidence, consistent results
- Good evidence, conflicting results
- Insufficient or absent evidence

TRANSLATION

Step 12: Determine fit, feasibility, and appropriateness of recommendation(s) for translation path.
Step 13: Create action plan.
Step 14: Secure support and resources to implement action plan.
Step 15: Implement action plan.
Step 16: Evaluate outcomes.
Step 17: Report outcomes to stakeholders.
Step 18: Identify next steps.
Step 19: Disseminate finding.

© 2017 The Johns Hopkins Hospital/Johns Hopkins University School of Nursing

Appendix 5.1

PET MANAGEMENT GUIDE

Initial EBP Question:						
EBP Team Leader(s):						
EBP Team Members:						
Activities	**Start Date**	**Days Required**	**End Date**	**Person Assigned**	**Milestone**	**Comment/ Resources Required**
PRACTICE QUESTION:						
Step 1: Recruit interprofessional team						
Step 2: Define the problem						
Step 3: Develop and refine the EBP question						
Step 4: Identify stakeholders						
Step 5: Determine responsibility for project leadership						
Step 6: Schedule team meetings						
EVIDENCE:						
Step 7: Conduct internal and external search for evidence						

(continued)

Activities	Start Date	Days Required	End Date	Person Assigned	Milestone	Comment/ Resources Required
Step 8: Appraise the level and quality of each piece of evidence						
Step 9: Summarize the individual evidence						
Step 10: Synthesize overall strength and quality of evidence						
Step 11: Develop recommendations for change based on evidence synthesis: • Strong, compelling evidence, consistent results • Good evidence, consistent results • Good evidence, conflicting results • Insufficient or absent evidence						
TRANSLATION:						
Step 12: Determine fit, feasibility, and appropriateness of recommendation(s) for translation path						
Step 13: Create action plan						
Step 14: Secure support and resources to implement action plan						

(continued)

Activities	Start Date	Days Required	End Date	Person Assigned	Milestone	Comment/ Resources Required
Step 15: Implement action plan						
Step 16: Evaluate outcomes						
Step 17: Report outcomes to stakeholders						
Step 18: Identify next steps						
Step 19: Disseminate findings						

© 2017 The Johns Hopkins Hospital/ Johns Hopkins University School of Nursing

6

Utilizing Data and Quality Improvement Principles

Janice Wilcox

"Quality needs to be constantly improved, but it is just as necessary to make sure that quality never deteriorates."
~Shigeru Mizuno

INTRODUCTION

Evidence demonstrates the value that clinical nurse leaders (CNLs) bring to healthcare by improving outcomes in many different areas. Some of these successes include decreasing falls, decreasing ventilator-associated pneumonia, reducing cancellations of surgical procedures, improving communication and rounding processes, and enhancing the patient satisfaction score (Bender, Connelly, Glaser, & Brown, 2012; L'Ecuyer, Shatto, Hoffman, & Crecelius, 2016; Phillips, Swiger, Flores, Clutter, & Reineck, 2012). These are only a few of the improvements that CNLs have made to organizations, as there many other areas where CNLs bring value to their microsystems. In order to improve processes and enhance care, CNLs must have knowledge of how to utilize data and quality improvement (QI) practices. Improvements do not occur without proper analysis and implementation of change. This chapter provides an overview of obtaining and utilizing data while utilizing QI principles and tools.

After reading this chapter, you will be able to:

1. Describe processes in sustaining high-reliability and value-based organizations
2. Recognize QI frameworks
3. Examine the use of data prior to and throughout the QI process
4. Identify common QI tools used during process improvement projects

TODAY'S HEALTHCARE ORGANIZATIONS

The Institute of Medicine (IOM) developed six aims for healthcare quality, which consist of care that is safe, timely, effective, efficient, equitable, and patient centered (STEEEP; Agency for Healthcare Research and Quality [AHRQ], 2018). However, high-quality care is not being achieved in a consistent manner throughout all healthcare organizations. The IOM (2007) noted that QI is of great importance in advancing healthcare and called for a greater emphasis on processes that improve value and the patient experience. These aims have created a climate within today's healthcare organizations that emphasize the need for improvement of practices and processes. Current practices within healthcare organizations are to ensure maintenance of value-based purchasing ideals and high-reliability processes. High-reliability organizations (HROs) refer to those entities that strive for improved reliability of practices, while intervening quickly when faults or errors occur (Latney, 2016). HROs not only seek to improve practices but also lookout for problems so they can be addressed before harm to the organization or patients occurs.

Value-based purchasing is also playing a major role in mandating safe practices. Value-based purchasing evolved from the high cost of healthcare, and the Centers for Medicare and Medicaid Services (CMS) quest to curtail those costs. Instead of fee for service reimbursement frameworks, where providers and organizations are paid according to the number of patients seen, the CMS is now reimbursing on the quality of services that patients receive. The CNL plays a major role in maintaining safe practice and HRO philosophies by utilizing their skill set of assessing systems for gaps in processes. It is essential to continuously assess and monitor processes to ensure practices are safe, current, and evidence based. The safer the practices are, the less likely the patients will be harmed, which improves the organization's bottom line. CNLs must be familiar with and use QI practices and tools to ensure safety and quality of care.

Essential Facts

Just as knowing and utilizing policy is critical to providing great patient care, understanding and applying QI principles is imperative when striving for successful, sustainable practice change.

QUALITY IMPROVEMENT

Healthcare organizations have been behind other areas of business and industry in utilizing QI principles but are now becoming more engaged in these practices due to the need to improve care. QI is defined by the Quality and Safety Education for Nurses Institute (QSEN) (2019) as the "use [of] data to monitor the outcomes of care processes and use [of] improvement methods to design and test changes to continuously improve the quality and safety of health care systems" (QSEN, 2019, table 4). Some consider QI to be both an art and a science in that questioning and developing ideas in addressing problems utilizes a creative and innovative mindset, whereas science enters into the process when utilizing improvement frameworks and analyzing results (D'Eramo, Davis, & Puckett, 2018). When working on QI initiatives, the team must have a clear idea of what the end product should be, or what is to be accomplished, as well as what the outcome will look like in order to know if goals have been reached. This process requires teamwork in identifying innovative means of addressing the issue and utilization of QI frameworks, principles, and techniques to attain positive results.

QI FRAMEWORKS

There are many QI frameworks that can assist the CNL when looking to improve care, but this chapter reviews a few of the most commonly seen in healthcare.

Donabedian

One of the first frameworks used in healthcare is the Donabedian model of quality assurance. Avedis Donabedian developed this model over 50 years ago and had profound insight into what was involved in creating quality healthcare. He proposed that quality in healthcare should be effective, efficient, acceptable, legitimate, and equitable, which coincides with current expert views (Donabedian, 2003). The healthcare components speak to science and technology improving practices and ensuring that improvements are efficient in utilizing resources, while also being sustainable. Donabedian also proposed that healthcare professionals consider the patient's wishes and values when determining care, which coincides with current evidence-based practice frameworks.

Essential Facts

Avedis Donabedian proposed the use of evidence garnered from a combination of science, patients, and practice years before the phrase *evidence-based practice* became widely used.

In order to ensure that these elements were embedded in processes of care, Donabedian developed a method of assessing environments of care using the structure, process, and outcome model.

Structure refers to "conditions under which care is provided" such as materials or equipment utilized (supplies, equipment, finances, informatics), people (medical, nursing, and ancillary staffing levels and clinical expertise), and characteristics of the organization (rural, urban, academic medical center; Donabedian, 2003, p. 46).

Process refers to "activities that constitute care—including diagnosis, treatment, rehabilitation, prevention, and patient education" (Donabedian, 2003, p. 46). Processes may include policies, reimbursement methods, and even the environment. They may also delve into how each part interacts, such as relationships between team members and patients, and coordination of care and educational services.

Outcomes refer to "changes (desirable or undesirable) in individuals and populations that can be attributed to healthcare" (Donabedian, 2003, p. 46). Note that the outcomes that are considered relate directly to patients and not the system. Every system outcome should therefore benefit the patient. Outcomes may consist of patient health, knowledge, behaviors, and satisfaction (Donabedian, 2003). The 5P (purpose, patients, professionals, processes, and patterns) assessment process that many CNLs learn to use in their programs of study coincides nicely with Donabedian model and can be very useful in identifying the structure, processes, and outcomes that Donabedian outlines.

Deming—Plan, Do, Study, Act

William Edwards Deming was a pioneer in QI and a leader in improving processes in the industrial world. He emphasized the need for better designs of services that would lead to high-level quality systems and developed the Plan, Do, Study, Act cycle, known by some as the Deming cycle. This model assists in gaining information and knowledge to continuously improve processes, products, or services (The W. Edwards Deming Institute, 2019).

Essential Facts

Deming cautions, "Stamping out fires is a lot of fun, but it is only putting things back the way they were" (The W. Edwards Deming Institute, 2019). This encourages CNLs to continue on toward the root of a problem instead of coming up with temporary solutions only.

The *Plan* begins with identifying a goal or purpose related to what is attempting to be accomplished. This requires a team to develop clear goals, measurable outcomes, and a vision of how the system will look once improved. This may be related to a rise in infection rates on a unit, and the goal would be to decrease those rates as evidenced by a decrease over the next 3 months.

The *Do* phase consists of carrying out the prescribed plan and collecting data on results. The plan may have been to educate nursing staff on the care of patients with catheter lines. Data collection would involve observing nurses to ensure adherence to policy and looking at data to determine if infection rates are decreasing.

The *Study* phase analyzes the progress of the plan to determine if success occurred and if there has been an impact on the outcomes. Criteria to determine impact may be as follows: Is there a decrease in infection rates? Is the decrease significant? or Should further actions be taken to address the problem, or should the plan continue?

During the *Act* phase, a determination is made as to whether the results are satisfactory, if the process should continue, or if adjustments are needed. If nurses are adhering to policy and infection rates continue to decrease, then the plan should continue. If infection rates remain high, the cycle should continue, and reevaluation of the plan should occur.

Lean Six Sigma/DMAIC

Lean Six Sigma was developed by the manufacturing industry as a means of increasing productivity, while at the same time maintaining product quality. Lean refers to eliminating waste while optimizing processes (Ha et al., 2016). Methods involve examination of processes and analyzing for defects in order to repair or eliminate faulty processes. Lean Six Sigma has been used to improve patient wait times in ambulatory settings, reducing the transfer of patients out of intensive care units, improve operating room efficiencies, and reduce hospital lengths of stay, along with other similar initiatives (Montella et al., 2017).

Lean Six Sigma integrates the DMAIC (define, measure, analyze, improve, control) steps to analyze and problem-solve healthcare setting concerns and issues (D'Eramo et al., 2018). During the define phase, a team is created to move through the problem-solving steps. The define phase is when the team works to develop a problem and goal statement, and a team or project charter is established. The charter is a document that describes and outlines the timeframe of work and the expected outcome. Process maps are generally used as a means of visualizing the different aspects of the problem and the expected deliverables (D'Eramo & Puckett, 2018).

During the measure phase, the current processes are examined, and variances are identified. The variances become the focus of the project in either eliminating or altering those processes, which cause the variance to improve the overall system. This is accomplished by analyzing data. Pareto charts and flowcharts are often used as a means of analyzing the frequency and the potential causes of the variance. These tools are discussed further in the following text. The measure phase then determines the variances, whereas the analyze phase determines the causes or why the variances are occurring. A root cause analysis may be performed to determine actual system flaws. Once the cause is determined, the improve phase begins by team members brainstorming potential solutions to address the problem. Once a solution is proposed, it is pilot-tested and further analyzed to determine its effectiveness. If the solution is found to be beneficial in addressing the original problem and is cost-effective, the practice is then adopted. The control phase works to sustain the change by continuing to monitor and measure results. These phases also include employee engagement of the change through standard change process means.

Essential Facts

Unlike some other QI frameworks, the control phase of Lean methodologies specifically encourages QI teams to drill down to the basic metrics they will need to continually observe and maintain change, as well as improve the intervention further (GoLeanSixSigma.com, n.d.).

ROOT CAUSE ANALYSIS

A root cause analysis is a method of retroactively determining the cause of an event or problem. This process is usually performed within a group and often performed by an interprofessional team. Steps of a root cause analysis consist of the following:

a. Determining what occurred
b. Determining what should have occurred
c. Determining causes of the event or contributing factors
d. Identifying root causes
e. Designing changes to eliminate the root cause
f. Measure to ensure continuous engagement of procedures (CMS, n.d-b.)

An example can be seen when two new graduate nurses, recently out of orientation, received orders to administer IV magnesium sulfate to their patients for low magnesium levels. Instead of the patients receiving their dosages over several hours, both patients received boluses of the medication in error. In examining the causes of these errors, it was determined that when setting up the tubing into the IV pump, both nurses inadvertently bypassed the pump causing the patients to receive boluses instead of a standard drip over time. This, however, is not the root cause of the problem; these are contributing factors to the overall problem. A team must examine the root causes of why two new nurses, on two different units, made the same mistake. In examining the process further, it was determined that the nurses were not totally familiar with the IV pump and how to administer IV piggy backs. Upon further review, it was determined that the nursing orientation provided a review of equipment but did not ensure nurse competence. The orientation educators felt competence was achieved on the unit level, and the unit educators assumed that competence was performed in general orientation. There was an overall misunderstanding about which educators were responsible for different forms of orientation. The recommended process change by the group was to redesign orientation to ensure nurses had oversight on use of patient care equipment within the unit where they were being precepted. This process change helped to alleviate that problem with this error, but further actions were necessary to ensure that there was a collaborative relationship between unit and general orientation educators. This example shows how important it is to really delve into the root cause and not stop at what the root cause appears to be.

5 Whys

Another useful method of determining root causes is the 5 Whys process. This method is quick and easy to use and allows relationships between different root causes to be identified. Each question should prompt another question until the actual root cause is determined (Centers for Medicare and Medicaid Services [CMS], n.d-a.) In the previous example of nurses administering magnesium sulfate, the team would ask the following:

1. Why did the patient receive a bolus? Answer: The nurses incorrectly threaded the IV tubing passing the IV pump when connecting the piggyback IV tubing.
2. Why did the nurses thread the tubing incorrectly? Answer: They were not familiar with the equipment.
3. Why were the nurses not familiar with the equipment? Answer: Orientation provided an overview of the equipment but did not include a competency check.
4. Why did orientation provide an overview and not ensure competence? Answer: There was a misunderstanding of processes between the organizational educators and unit educators.
5. Why was there a misunderstanding between educators? Answer: They did not collaborate on educational processes (CMS, n.d-a.).

As noted in this example, the 5 Whys can be very beneficial in analyzing patient errors and gaps in system processes.

Essential Facts

Using the 5 Whys in conjunction with the root cause analysis framework can be a particularly effective combination when attempting to identify a problem's origin and find a reasonable solution.

Failure Mode Effects Analysis

Failure mode and effects analysis (FMEA) is a structured method of determining potential failures or problems within a system. The process attempts to identify "all the ways a process could fail [and] estimate the probability and consequences of each failure" (Finkelman, 2018, p. 366). The process identifies ways in which a failure could occur and attempts to prevent the failure from occurring. This is accomplished through the development of a team to answer three questions.

1. What could go wrong?

2. Why would the failures occur?
3. What would be the consequences of each failure? (D'Eramo et al., 2018, p. 404).

When analyzing systems and processes, identification of hazards such as human factors, equipment failures, and environmental factors can all be potential risks that may lead to errors or harm. When potential risks are identified, the team will then work to address them by prioritizing actions based on degree of potential risks (D'Eramo et al., 2018).

If the FMEA method was used in the previous example of the new nurses and the IV piggyback administration, the errors may not have occurred. The FMEA process would have allowed identification of the potential risk when asking what could go wrong when a new nurse administered IV medications. The answer could have been that the nurse may not thread the IV tubing correctly. Why would the failures occur would be answered by the nurses not having sufficient knowledge of the equipment. The potential consequences would be significant as the error could cause patient harm or even death. This would be a high priority risk since it may involve a sentinel patient event.

CNLs can find each of these QI models useful in identifying and addressing problems, gaps, and concerns within the microsystem. Many organizations have experienced leaders who oversee QI processes and who can assist and mentor CNLs in becoming familiar with techniques to improve processes. An aspect of QI that needs to be considered along with the type of QI methodology used is having the correct data to communicate the need for further investigation and potential change. CNLs are very good at identifying problems within the microsystem, but it is the data that will gain attention from stakeholders and help communicate the need for further interventions to be initiated.

Essential Facts

The CNL roles of risk anticipator and systems analyst must be initiated early and implemented fully in order to lead the microsystem through effective QI activities.

DATA COLLECTION AND ANALYSIS

Sources and Types of Data

Data are the raw numbers that measure processes and outcomes (D'Eramo & Puckett, 2018, p. 418) and are used to "identify potential quality concerns and describe problems, gaps, trends, patterns, and so on" (Finkelman, 2018, p. 336). Data can be quantitative or qualitative and primary or secondary. Quantitative data are numerical information that can be counted, measured, and analyzed through statistical measures. Quantitative data can be used to determine specific outcomes such as length of stay, readmissions, or number of hospital-acquired conditions. Quantitative data will also be the data used to determine if a QI project is actually improving processes. Qualitative data describe something and are often gathered from surveys or questionnaires or through one-on-one discussion. This type of data may be useful in gathering information on how patients feel about certain aspects of care, such as their providers or care team. Both types of data can be useful in determining gaps and improving processes, but quantitative data will provide the numbers that show the impact of a problem or improvement.

Essential Facts

Four main quantitative research designs include descriptive, correlational, quasi-experimental, and experimental. Three common qualitative research designs include phenomenology, grounded theory, and ethnography (Information Resources Management Association, 2015).

Data can be obtained from a number of sources depending upon the problem or initiative. Primary data are data that are collected for a specific purpose or project that you may be working on. For example, if you are executing an intervention to improve staff satisfaction, you would collect specific data to determine if the intervention improved staff satisfaction. Surveys may be used to ask specific questions using numeric rating scores to determine the degree of improvement. Secondary data are data that were initially obtained for another purpose. An example of secondary data is patient information within the electronic medical record (EMR) that was collected for patient care purposes. This type of data can be useful for QI initiatives, especially when it pertains to patient outcomes such as hospital-acquired conditions, readmissions, and length of stay problems (Johnson & Sylvia, 2018). The EMR can provide information on demographics, administrative data such as insurance coverage, charges for services, practitioner services provided, health risks and health status, medical history, medical management, and outcomes data.

There are many different sources of data besides the EMR that may include other databases within the individual organization, state and regional hospital organizations, departments of health, and federal agencies (AHRQ, 2016). Organizations usually maintain certain dashboards consisting of charts and graphs, which provide an overview of quality indicators. The healthcare cost and utilization project (HCUP) provides inpatient and outpatient discharge information from private and federal entities and state and hospital organizations and can be found at http://hcupnet.ahrq.gov/. The Medicare Provider Analysis and Review (MEDPAR) is a database collected from all Medicare beneficiaries who have utilized inpatient hospital and skilled nursing facilities. Since this is a Medicare database, the data generally consist of information for older populations (AHRQ, 2016). The MEDPAR database can be found at https://www.cms.gov/Research-Statistics-Data-and-Systems/Statistics-Trends-and-Reports/MedicareFeeforSvcPartsAB/MEDPAR. Data from the National Database of Nursing Quality can also be beneficial for some types of QI initiatives, and reports are often distributed to organizations on a regular basis. The Centers for Disease Control and Prevention provides data on incidence and prevalence of certain communicable diseases and conditions and can be found at cdc.gov/datastatistics/index.html. Hospital benchmark information can be found at the Medicare Hospital Compare Data site at data.medicare.gov. These are just a few of the data sources available to nurses involved in QI projects.

Data Collection and Analysis of a QI Project

When initiating a QI project, it is important to have a well-developed plan in order to determine if the project is meeting established goals. First and foremost, a team should be compiled to develop project goals and to determine data sources used for collecting relevant data to determine if goals are being met. It is also important that those involved in the collection of data understand the process of collecting data, especially if certain tools or surveys will be used.

When collecting data to determine if a QI project is resulting in the desired outcomes, it is important to consider reliability and validity of the tools. Reliability refers to the "competence of the data collection mechanism to *consistently measure what it is intended to measure*" (Johnson & Sylvia, 2018, p. 71). Validity refers to the degree to which a measure is actually measuring what it is intended to measure (Finkelman, 2018; Johnson & Sylvia, 2018). For example, if a survey is to measure staff satisfaction regarding a particular aspect of their work, the survey must have been previously evaluated to ensure its validity in measuring staff satisfaction and reliability in consistently measuring staff satisfaction levels. It is often beneficial to search for studies that have used the specific tools to ensure they are reliable and valid.

It is also important to ensure interrater reliability if there is more than one individual collecting data (Johnson & Sylvia, 2018). This means that all data collectors are following the same guidelines and asking questions in the same manner to ensure validity of collected data. Interrater reliability can be determined by observing data collectors while they are using tools or methods of data collection. It is also very important to educate the data collectors on procedures prior to initiation of the data collection process.

The QI project plan should include identification of the following:

- What is being measured (e.g., infection rates)?
- Where and how the data will be obtained (e.g., EMR)?
- The total population of interest (denominator) (e.g., a particular medical surgical unit)
- The subpopulation (numerator) (e.g., patients developing hospital acquired infections)
- Determining data collection procedures and who will collect the data
- A project timeline (Finkelman, 2018)

For example, you are the CNL on a general medical unit who has seen an increase in hospital-acquired infection rates over the past 3 months; 10% of the population or 10 patients out of 100 developed a hospital-acquired infection. You developed a new evidence-based QI initiative to address this problem and compiled a team of unit nurses to assist in educating the staff and monitor data for potential improvement. Your goal is to decrease the infection rates by 50% over the next 3 months. Therefore, the "what you will be measuring" is the hospital-acquired infection rates over the next 3 months. Your population is the patients on your particular unit, and the subpopulation would be those patients who have developed a hospital-acquired infection during that timeframe (this will be important when analyzing the data). Data will be collected by you and another nurse from the EMR during the next 3 months, which is your timeline. (This timeline is to simplify this example; in reality, you would want to compile data more often and assess staff compliance with the process, as well as the patient outcome data.) At the end of the 3 months, your data from the EMR showed that 5 out of 100 patients or 5% of the population developed a hospital-acquired infection. The goal of your project was to decrease the infection rate by 50%, and in calculating the difference, you reached your goal. This example is simplistic but provides an overview of the process of data collection and analysis.

> **Essential Facts**
>
> CNLs need to equate QI results to financial savings. For example, a reduced pressure ulcer rate is great, but what does that mean in dollars and cents? (Cost of additional care for a pressure ulcer, $43,180 according to Medicare) × (Number of pressure ulcers in a certain time period) = Total cost of pressure ulcers. Performing this equation pre- and postintervention will provide the evidence of savings.

QI TOOLS

There are a number of tools that can assist in describing and analyzing data as well as processes that can help guide QI initiatives. Utilization of these tools will permit easy identification and interpretation of data.

Cause and Effect Diagrams

Cause and effect diagrams are also known as fishbone diagrams because they resemble the bones of a fish. These diagrams are useful in identifying root causes and contributing factors associated with a problem. The problem is placed in a box on the right side or "head" of the fish. Organizational categories are listed, and below each of these categories, primary and secondary causes are listed. Common categories that can be considered for headings include equipment, environment, people, processes, materials, methods, and equipment materials, as it is under these headings that primary and secondary causes of problems occur and can be listed. The primary causes are written on the horizontal arrows, and the secondary causes are listed diagonally from the primary arrows (Institute for Healthcare Improvement [IHI], 2017).

Pareto Charts

Pareto charts are based on the premise that 80% of problems are caused by 20% of issues within the organization. The chart permits visualization of those major concerns that contribute to the issues being addressed. The pareto chart is basically a bar graph that assists in easily visualizing causes and frequency of problems. It allows data to be seen in a hierarchical manner with the most significant problems on the left of the chart visualized by taller bars and the less significant causes to the right of the graph. Utilizing this tool allows a quality team to determine problems that are the most significant and, therefore, considered to be the priority in addressing as the team moves forward in developing initiatives (American Society for Quality, 2019).

Run Charts

Run charts depict data over a period of time, which helps to determine trends and patterns in workflows or processes. This tool is very good at looking at whether or not processes are stable or if there are large tendencies of variance. It permits a quick and easy analysis of whether a process is working as intended. There is a median line within the chart, and if data points are located close to the median, consistency of processes exists. If data points are spread out at different points within the graph, variance in processes is occurring and usually signifies problems or potential problems in the process (D'Eramo & Puckett, 2018).

Flowcharts

Flowcharts are a great tool in looking at processes such as patient flows, workflows, and processes. These charts allow visualization of each step of a process and permit all parties to see where they fit within a particular workflow or patient flow throughout the system. It can also alert teams to variances, waste, delays, and inefficiencies. Flowcharts are created using different symbols; an oval is generally used for the beginning and end of a process with other symbols being used for activities, decision points, wait, or delays. Arrows are used for directional purposes showing such things as how a patient moves throughout the system. It is best to begin the chart with the beginning and end and filling in the processes in the middle. These charts are usually kept simple but can become more elaborate depending upon the process (IHI, 2017).

Gantt Charts

Gantt charts are used as a means of managing an overall improvement project. These charts help in planning, organizing, and tracking certain tasks along the way. These are a useful tool in tracking progress of the different tasks or steps that need to be completed and allow the team to stay on track by reviewing and updating throughout the QI project. These are also beneficial in stimulating the group to continue, as they permit visualization of what has actually been accomplished.

These are just a few of the many charts and graphs that can be applied to data and project improvement initiatives. The IHI has a

> **Clinical Nurse Leader Vignette 6.1:**
> **Decreasing Supply Waste in a Surgical Intensive Care Unit**
>
> A frequently mentioned administrative problem within a surgical intensive care unit was the cost of supplies. Marcy, the CNL on the unit, identified there was a waste of unused supplies brought into the patient's room during the patient stay. The supplies were being discarded when the patient was transferred out of the unit. Marcy was familiar with Lean QI techniques and understood that these techniques had been successful in other industries in reducing waste. She also understood that nurses did not always understand their roles in decreasing wasteful practices and the impact it may have on the unit and overall organization. Marcy began her project by consulting with the infection prevention department to ensure that unused supplies that had not come in contact with the patient could be returned for use by other patients and was informed that this was an acceptable practice.
>
> Her interventions focused on increasing awareness of supply cost and initiating a system to recycle supplies by placing bins in each patient room to collect unused supplies to be returned to the supply room upon patient discharge. Marcy developed a survey for staff to determine their awareness of supply costs and habits regarding supply usage and collected items that were to be discarded after a patient's discharge and totaled the cost of the items. She then created a poster indicating the waste of supplies, cost, and impact of the waste on the unit and organization. Each supply cubicle in the supply room was labeled with prices. Several in-services were held to educate the staff on the problem and the new initiative. To ensure change would occur on the unit, Marcy provided real-time feedback, fostered a sense of shared responsibility for the change, and initiated a reward program. After the project had been in place for 10 months, surveys indicated an improved sense of knowledge of cost and waste by staff and a 96% reduction in supply waste. The initiative was so successful that administration planned to replicate the initiative on other units.

document that outlines many of the more popular QI tools and can be found at www.ihi.org/resources/Pages/Tools/Quality-Improvement-Essentials-Toolkit.aspx. There are also many YouTube tutorials available on creating many of these charts.

References

Agency for Healthcare Research and Quality. (2016). *Databases used for hospital quality measures.* Retrieved from https://www.ahrq.gov/talkingquality/measures/setting/hospitals/databases.html

Agency for Healthcare Research and Quality. (2018). *Six domains of health care quality.* Retrieved from https://www.ahrq.gov/talkingquality/measures/six-domains.html

American Society for Quality. (2019). *Learn about quality. What is a Pareto chart?* Retrieved from https://asq.org/quality-resources/pareto

Bender, M., Connelly, C. D., Glaser, D., & Brown, C. (2012). Clinical nurse leader impact on microsystem care quality. *Nursing Research, 61,* 326–332. doi:10.1097/NNR.0b013e318265a5b6

Centers for Medicare and Medicaid Services. (n.d.-a). *Five whys for RCA tool.* Retrieved from https://www.cms.gov/Medicare/Provider-Enrollment-and-Certification/QAPI/downloads/FiveWhys.pdf

Centers for Medicare and Medicaid Services. (n.d.-b). *Guidance for performing root cause analysis (RCA) with performance improvement projects (PIPs).* Retrieved from www.cms.gov/medicare/provider-enrollment-and-certification/qapi/downloads/guidanceforrca.pdf

D'Eramo, A. L., Davis, M., & Puckett, J. B. (2018). Essentials of quality improvement. In P. Kelly, B. A. Vottero, & C. A. Christie-McAuliffe (Eds.), *Introduction to quality and safety education for nurses. Core competencies for nursing leadership and management* (2nd ed., pp. 375–416). New York, NY: Springer Publishing Company.

D'Eramo, A. L., & Puckett, J. B. (2018). Tools of quality improvement. In P. Kelly, B. A. Vottero, & C. A. Christie-McAuliffe (Eds.), *Introduction to quality and safety education for nurses. Core competencies for nursing leadership and management* (2nd ed., pp. 417–445). New York, NY: Springer Publishing Company.

Donabedian, A. (2003). *An introduction to quality assurance in health care.* New York, NY: Oxford University Press, Inc.

Finkelman, A. (2018). *Quality improvement. A guide for integration in nursing.* Burlington, MA: Jones and Bartlett Learning.

GoLeanSixSigma. (n.d.). *Control—Phase 5 (of 5) of Lean Six Sigma.* Retrieved from https://goleansixsigma.com/control-phase-5-of-5-of-lean-six-sigma/

Ha, C., McCoy, D. A., Taylor, C. B., Kirk, K. D., Fry, R. S., & Modi, J. R. (2016). Using Lean Six Sigma methodology to improve a mass immunizations process at the United States naval academy. *Military Medicine, 181*(6), 582–588. doi:10.7205/MILMED-D-15-00247

Information Resources Management Association. (2015). *Research methods: Concepts, methodologies, tools, and applications.* Hershey, PA: IGI Global.

Institute for Healthcare Improvement. (2017). *QI essentials toolkit*. Retrieved from http://www.ihi.org/resources/Pages/Tools/Quality-Improvement-Essentials-Toolkit.aspx

The Institute of Medicine. (2007). *The state of quality improvement and implementation research: Expert views*. Washington, DC: National Academies Press.

Johnson, E., & Sylvia, M. L. (2018). Secondary data collection. In M. L. Sylvia & M. F. Terhaar (Eds.), *Clinical analytics and data management for the DNP* (2nd ed., pp. 61–86). New York, NY: Spring Publishing Company.

Latney, C. R. (2016). The need for a paradigm shift in healthcare culture: Old versus new. In C. A. Oster & J. S. Braaten (Eds.), *High reliability organizations. A healthcare handbook for patient safety and quality.* (pp. 4–24). Indianapolis, IN: Sigma Theta Tau International.

L'Ecuyer, K. M., Shatto, B. J., Hoffman, R. L., & Crecelius, M. L. (2016). The certified clinical nurse leader in critical care. *Dimensions of Critical Care Nursing, 35*(5), 248–254. doi:10.1097/DCC.0000000000000202

Montella, E., Di Cicco, M. V., Ferraro, A., Raiola, E., Triassi, M., Centobelli, P., & Improta, G. (2017). The application of Lean Six Sigma methodology to reduce the risk of healthcare-associated infections in surgery departments. *Journal of Evaluation in Clinical Practice, 23*(3), 530–539. doi:10.1111/jep.12662

Phillips, S., Swiger, P. A., Flores, R., Clutter, P., & Reineck, C. (2012). Clinical nurse leader: Emerging role to optimize unit level performance. *The Army Medical Department Journal*, 77–83.

QSEN Institute. (2019). *Graduate KSAs: Quality improvement*. Retrieved from http://qsen.org/competencies/graduate-ksas/#quality_improvement

The W. Edwards Deming Institute. (2019). *PDSA cycle*. Retrieved from https://deming.org/explore/p-d-s-a

Coordination of Care

Janice Wilcox

"When 'I' is replaced with 'we' even illness becomes wellness."
~Malcolm X

INTRODUCTION

Coordination of care activities is listed throughout the Competencies and Curricular Expectations for the Clinical Nurse Leader Education and Practice (American Association of Colleges of Nursing [AACN], 2013) and is emphasized within the formal education of the clinical nurse leader (CNL). These competencies include such things as leading interprofessional teams in delivering patient-centered care, evaluating handoffs and transitions of care, facilitating lateral integration of care across the continuum of care, and utilizing coaching skills in assisting individuals in the management of their own care (AACN, 2013). The CNL is, therefore, educated on these practices and instrumental in ensuring that coordination of services is accomplished. This knowledge is greatly needed within healthcare systems to improve gaps that are present that lead to duplication of services, hospital readmissions, increased morbidity and mortality rates, along with other patient and healthcare problems. This chapter highlights major gaps in care coordination and transitioning of care and provides measures for the CNL to use to improve coordination processes.

After reading this chapter, you will be able to:

1. Define care coordination
2. Recognize transition of care models
3. Identify challenges and strategies of care coordination
4. Analyze the impact of health literacy and social determinants of health on coordination of care

COORDINATION OF CARE

Coordination of care is considered of great importance within healthcare organizations and healthcare agencies. The Centers for Medicare and Medicaid Services (CMS) recently initiated *Bundled Payments for Care Improvement Advanced* as a means of improving coordination of care (CMS, 2018). The National Quality Forum (NQF) and the Agency for Healthcare Research and Quality (AHRQ) have both made coordination of care initiatives priorities and created reports providing insights and suggestions to improve quality of care along the continuum of care (McDonald et al., 2014; NQF, 2014). The American Nurses Association (ANA) has reported on the importance of the registered nurse in achieving coordination outcomes in several publications (ANA, 2012; Lamb, 2013; Lamb & Newhouse, 2018).

The rationale for these organizations and agencies making care coordination a priority is because of the many improved outcomes that are seen from effective practices in this area. Care coordination activities have been especially helpful for the elderly and those patients with multiple comorbidities. Overall, improved outcomes have been noted in the following areas:

- Decreased utilization of ED facilities
- Reductions in hospitalizations and readmissions
- Decreases in mortality rates and improved quality of life
- Improvement in functional ability of patients with chronic diseases
- Improved patient adherence to plans of care
- Reduction of overall healthcare costs
- Increased patient satisfaction (ANA, 2012; NQF, 2014)

However, the main reason for effective coordination of care is to create systems that improve the patient and family member's journey, as they move through complex and often confusing environments. Every healthcare professional will encounter the system at some point, as either a patient or a family member, and has the responsibility to care for each patient in the manner they themselves would desire. The CNL has a pivotal role in these processes.

DEFINING COORDINATION OF CARE

There is no one definition of coordination of care, as each discipline and agency defines coordination of care slightly differently. However, key characteristics are found within these definitions. The NQF (2014) defines it as "a function that helps ensure that the patient's needs and preferences for health services and information sharing across people, functions, and sites are met over time" (p. 5). Lamb (2013) states that care coordination is "the 'glue' of our healthcare system, the process that transpires between patients, families, and members of the healthcare team to organize care and assure that everyone and every service is aligned and working toward the same goal" (p. 3). Organizations differ in how they manage coordination of care, and many have a coordination team that may include nursing case managers, utilization review nurses, social workers, and perhaps even pharmacists. These professionals manage the care and determine what care and resources the patient will need moving throughout the system.

Essential Facts

The need for care coordination was born out of the healthcare progression from single primary care physicians managing an individual through the care continuum to interdisciplinary teams collaborating to provide holistic care to patients across settings.

The CNL is a much-needed resource to the team since CNLs are knowledgeable about the particular population of patient within their microsystem and understand what may be required in the way of services to ensure smooth transitioning within or outside of the organization. The CNL coordinates care within the microsystem by, first and foremost, connecting with patients and families to understand their priorities and concerns. Other CNL activities include educating and guiding staff and communicating with care team members. The communication involves ensuring that every aspect of the patient's care within the care setting, discharge strategies, and transitions of care is included within the plan of care. The CNL and organizations may be able to enhance coordination strategies by adopting a particular transition of care model to guide them through coordination activities.

TRANSITION OF CARE MODELS

A variety of evidence-based models exist, and a listing of a few with web links can be found in Table 7.1. Each model addresses transitioning of patients in different ways. Depending upon your area of practice and the focus of your facility, one model may work better than another.

The Project Boost Model focuses on hospital readmission and was developed by the Society of Hospitalists. The main goal of this model is to improve discharge processes through utilization of multidisciplinary teams and mentors. There are a variety of tools that are based on quality improvement principles that aid in the process.

The Care Transitions Intervention® (CTI) utilizes a transitions coach who assists the patient through the transition process. The model is based on four pillars: medication self-management, a patient-centered health record, primary care and specialist follow-up, and red flag recognition. The coach assists the patient in activities to improve self-care management (Enderlin et al., 2013; Sheikh et al., 2018).

The Guided Care Model was developed by The Johns Hopkins University and focuses on chronically ill patients by collaborating with primary care providers (PCPs) to provide more cost-effective, patient-centered care. This model utilizes a nurse as a guide to assist the patient throughout the transitions process through educational and coordination activates. There is also a focus on obtaining

Table 7.1

Transition of Care Models

Project Boost (Better Outcomes by Optimizing Safe Transitions)	www.hospitalmedicine.org
Care Transitions Interventions (CTI®)	https://caretransitions.org
Guided Care Model Comprehensive Primary Care for Complex Patients	http://guidedcare.org
Interventions to Reduce Acute Care Transfers (INTERACT®)	www.pathway-interact.com
Home Health Model of Care Transitions	http://ahhqi.org/images/uploads/AHHQI_Care_Transitions_Tools_Kit_r011314.pdf
Transitional Care Model	www.transitionalcare.info/
Chronic Care Model	www.improvingchroniccare.org/index.php?p=The_Chronic_CareModel&s=2

community services for patients in need (Enderlin et al., 2013; Sheikh et al., 2018).

The INTERACT® Model is mostly focused on healthcare professionals in extended care facilities (ECFs). This model provides tools and resources to educate professionals on early warning signs that help them in the assessment and evaluation phase of patients in order to treat prior to the need for hospitalization. The site offers many training opportunities and resources that may assist clinicians (Enderlin et al., 2013; Sheikh et al., 2018).

The Home Health Model of Care Transitions was also developed to address hospital readmissions but for patients in their own homes. The model is patient centric and focuses on medication management, community and care coordination, patient education, and coaching along with follow-up care from healthcare professionals outside of the hospital setting (Enderlin et al., 2013; Sheikh et al., 2018).

The Transitional Care Model (TCM) was created at the University of Pennsylvania as a means of preparing high-risk patients with multiple chronic conditions and their caregivers on self-care practices as a means of managing their many challenges. The ultimate goal is to reduce hospital readmission. This model utilizes a nurse as transitional coordinator who collaborates with the multidisciplinary care providers, makes home care visits, and assesses and educates patients in an attempt to enhance independence (Enderlin et al., 2013; Sheikh et al., 2018).

The Chronic Care Model (CCM) focuses on the management of chronic care conditions. This model looks at the interplay of the health systems—both acute and ambulatory settings. It examines the health system culture, decision support systems, and clinical information systems, along with community resources to determine if these processes enable the patient to become an active partner in the management of their conditions. It helps to identify areas that require modification to enhance services and outcomes (The Chronic Care Model, 2019; Enderlin, et al., 2013).

Essential Facts

Transition of care models support the second of the 10 Rules of Healthcare Redesign listed in Crossing the Quality Chasm: "Care is customized according to patient needs and values. The system should be designed to meet the most common types of needs, but should have the capability to respond to individual patient choices and preferences" (IOM, 2001).

ANALYZING READMISSIONS

CNLs are the experts when it comes to recognizing needs of their particular patient population, but the CNL must also analyze data to determine if unit and organizational processes are sufficient in managing multiple needs of patients. Readmission rates are a standard measurement of quality in most acute care organizations. The CNL must determine why patients are being readmitted and determine gaps in processes that may have prevented those readmissions. Common areas to assess are as follows: Was the patient discharged to home or a facility—if they were discharged to home, were home care services provided? What types of services were provided and were the services sufficient to meet the needs of the patient? Was the patient discharged to a skilled nursing facility (SNF) or ECF? Is there documentation from the home care agency, SNF, or ECF that can be reviewed to analyze why the patient's status declined causing the need for acute care admission? Are there patterns of readmission stemming from discharging patients to certain facilities or home care agencies? Should particular agencies or facilities be avoided in future discharge planning? Is there a relationship between the acute care facility and the SNF, ECF, and home care agencies to address readmission concerns? Was the patient educated on their illness or condition prior to discharge? Did the patient understand how to care for self and did they obtain follow-up care; if not why? What were the barriers for the patient in following their plan of care and obtaining follow-up care? Are community resources available for patients who are returning home? Are follow-up phone calls performed by a member of the acute care organization to ensure patient compliance and address additional barriers? Was the patient's plan of care adequate or were services from other disciplines omitted that would have been beneficial in addressing all of the patient's needs?

Essential Facts

Within the system analyst and outcomes manager roles, CNLs critically look beyond poor outcomes and dig for the root causes of process inefficiency and system failure, attempting to repair problems from their origin.

Answering these questions will stimulate the CNL's critical thinking in determining why the patient did not receive adequate services, why the SNF or ECF missed signs of patient decline leading to a readmission, why the patient was not educated or education was insufficient in leading to patient or caregiver understanding of self-care, what barriers existed for the patient in performing self-care measures, and what community resources were missed or lacking to meet all of the patient's needs. The answers then lead the CNL determining if organizational practices and referrals need to be improved and guide the search for best practice to address these gaps. In addition, when looking at the answers to these questions, the CNL should consider different challenges and strategies to enhance transitional planning and care that lead to improved outcomes for the patient and decrease readmissions to the acute care facility.

CHALLENGES AND STRATEGIES FOR COORDINATING CARE

Communication

Whether it is in coordination of care for patients within an organization or in transitioning the patient to outpatient or home services, communication is the greatest barrier. Handoff communication between departments, such as when a patient is transferred from the ED, is complicated. Handoffs usually involve communication between many disciplines, several departments, and nursing staff. Most nurses have dealt with lack of communication regarding a patient's condition, medications, and procedures, which leads to frustration for the nurse and gaps in care for the patient. Communication has been the focus of many quality improvement and safety initiatives for many years, which has led to the development and usage of SBAR (situation, background, assessment, recommendation) and CUS (concerned, uncomfortable, safety) tools to improve communication practices.

The CNL is instrumental in assessing and evaluating communication practices within the clinical setting to ensure accurate information is being transferred to every department. This can be done by analyzing gaps in processes that inhibit communication, ensuring that employees are taking time to complete SBAR documentation, which enhances accurate interdepartmental communication. It is also important for the CNL to oversee interdisciplinary communication and rounding, being the link for all stakeholders. Patients, families, and caregivers are often provided information from various healthcare professionals and may be given conflicting information from different disciplines. The CNL can diminish this fragmentation by being that "go to" person for patient's questions and answers. It is of great importance that the patient is included in conversations no matter whether the patient is moving within or outside of a particular organization.

Essential Facts

CNLs are trained to be master communicators, effective collaborators, and lateral integrators, contributing to the healthy work environment of any healthcare practice setting.

Communication is especially problematic when transitioning patients to care outside of the organization. Kerstenetzky, Birschbach, Beach, Hager, and Kennelty (2017) determined that SNFs and ECFs often found that discrepancies in orders occur when patients transferred from acute care settings and the patients are not always aware of their medications. Along with the discrepancies, personnel in these facilities found it difficult to contact hospital employees to answer questions. PCPs often find it difficult to determine the exact reason for admission and what exactly occurred during the hospitalization. An example of this can be seen when the hospitalist discharges a patient following hospitalization for a cerebral vascular accident (CVA). The diagnosis of CVA is communicated, but there was an omission in documentation that the underlying cause of the CVA was cocaine abuse (Rattray et al., 2017). The plan of care for this patient may be totally different from another patient suffering a CVA. The CNL can be the point person within the acute care facility to assist in the discharge and follow-up process. Whether patients are discharged to home or a facility, follow-up phone calls have been found to be very helpful in ensuring continuity and decreasing readmissions (Cloonan, Wood, & Riley, 2013). The CNL can enhance communication and lead in developing a standardized care transitions pathway that would include all pertinent discharge information that can be sent to facilities, home care agencies, PCPs, and even home with the patient. Utilization of one of the transitions of care models can be very helpful in improving communication.

Another communication issue is the electronic medical record (EMR). Many SNFs, ECFs, and PCPs find the discharge summaries confusing and difficult to find if they even have access to the same particular EMR (Rattray et al., 2017). Most of the acute care documentation is chronologically written, which makes it difficult for other care providers to find specific information from a particular discipline or clinical service. This may lead to further gaps in care, or delays in treatments, as there may not be sufficient time to read through the entire hospitalization to find specific information. Other issues with the EMR are the lack of ability to track priority patients in need of care coordination, such as chronic care patients, and inability to obtain reports to determine if care coordination activities have been completed and follow-up has occurred (Lamb & Newhouse, 2018). CNLs can be advocates for improved systems that permit communication across systems and better analytical programming. With this in mind, the CNL can collaborate with other healthcare professionals to determine their views on system deficiencies and work with informatics teams in developing improved analytical systems that would eventually improve transitional processes.

Patient-Centered Care

As stated previously, it is essential for CNLs to engage patients in their care and planning of their care. This is especially important when caring for chronic care patients with multiple comorbidities. When patients are seen by multiple care providers and are on numerous medications, fragmentation is especially concerning. Care that is considered patient centered is becoming more prevalent throughout organizations. In the past, care was directed by the desires of the physician and what the physician saw as priorities. Today, greater emphasis is being placed on engaging patients to determine goals, which is said to improve outcomes and decrease readmissions (Bucknall et al., 2016). The Institute of Medicine (2001) refers to patient-centered care as care that is safe, effective, timely, equitable, and efficient. Greene, Tuzzio, and Cherkin (2012) describe patient-centered care as "that which honors patients' preferences, needs and values; applies a biopsychological perspective rather than a purely biomedical perspective; and forges a strong partnership between patient and clinician" (p. 49).

For the CNL, a patient-centered care approach begins with the initiation of an empathetic, caring relationship with the patient, one who listens and considers the physical aspects of care along with the psychosocial aspects of care. The patient's family and caregivers are also important to engage, especially if the patient is unable to care for themselves. The information that follows concentrates on the patient, but inclusion of family can also be as important.

Patient-centered care involves engaging in active listening, where the nurse is hearing and processing what is being said and does not become distracted by other concerns. When talking to patients about their concerns, make sure to turn off phones and electronic devices, make eye contact, and sit facing the patient to provide an atmosphere of concern and caring. Also, be aware of nonverbal communication patterns, such as body position, gestures, and overall appearance, as these are important when attempting to convey interest and concern. Ask open-ended questions to engage the patient. Instead of asking "Are you feeling better today?" which prompts a yes or no answer, phrase the question as "How are you feeling today?" Another example would be stating "You seem upset about something today" instead of "Are you upset about something?" Avoid the use of "why" when talking with a patient. Asking why can elicit a defensive emotion within the patient.

Essential Facts

According to Brooks and John, four kinds of conversational questions include the following:
- Introductory questions ("How are you?")
- Mirror questions ("I'm fine. How are you?")
- Full-switch questions (ones that change the topic entirely)
- Follow-up questions (ones that solicit more information) (Brooks & John [2018], "Favor follow-up questions," para. 1)

Within patient-centered care frameworks of practice, it is important to understand what the patient's priorities are and what they are most concerned about. The patient must be an active participant in their care and be asked what is important to them, and how they feel they can manage their own healthcare needs. Using a shared decision-making approach can be helpful when determining the collaborative plan of care with the patient. Shared decision-making is about working the plan into the patient's daily life according to their own preferences. The Mayo Clinic https://shareddecisions.mayoclinic.org has many resources on shared decision-making such as describing the benefits and risks of taking statin medications to reduce the risk of a heart attack. The tool provides the number of people who have benefited from taking statins along with the potential risks associated with statin usage. This tool along with others permit the patient to understand the significance of the treatment along with downsides so they can make the decision.

Motivational interviewing can also be beneficial in assisting patients in goal setting. Motivational interviewing is a form of conversation that enhances a person's motivation and commitment to change (Katz, 2020). The nurse or other healthcare provider uses acceptance and compassion in engaging the patient to determine measures to perform that could improve their health status. Some suggest that healthcare professionals should be trained in the use of motivational interviewing skills, and training programs are available in many organizations. More information can be found at https://motivationalinterviewing.org.

When discussing care with the patient, it is also important to identify the patient's health literacy levels and understand how social determinants of health affect a person's ability to care for self. Healthcare professionals are quick to state that patients are noncompliant with treatment plans, but it is often the case that patients are not necessarily noncompliant by choice, but the noncompliance is due to extenuating circumstances.

Health Literacy

Health literacy deals with a person's ability to understand written and verbal health information. Cloonan et al. (2013) state that "approximately 36% of adults in the United States have limited literacy skills, and an additional 30 million adults have below basic skills" (p. 383). Low health literacy can lead to greater risk of rehospitalization and poorer health outcomes. This inability to understand healthcare information is a main cause of patient's not adhering to plans of care.

Essential Facts

It is critical that our patients understand the healthcare education provided to them. "Otherwise, we didn't reach them, and that is the same as if we didn't treat them" (Benjamin, 2010, p. 784).

Techniques that can enhance understanding are to ensure that each piece of written material is written at a fourth-grade reading level and conveys no more than three major points. Pictorial illustrations can be very beneficial in enhancing understanding. Verbal communication and teachings should be provided in a slow, non-rushed manner, limiting the use of any technical and medical terminology. The use of teach-back techniques, where the patient is asked to confirm what they have been told or instructed, assists nurses in determining comprehension and misunderstanding of information. Follow-up phone calls can be beneficial in reinforcing teaching if the patient has been discharged or seen in a primary care facility. Patients can forget easily, and the need for reinforcement is very important.

Social Determinants of Health

Social determinants of health include socioeconomic status, educational level, neighborhood or community in which a person resides, employment, social support, and access to care. These issues have a great bearing not only on provision of care but also on whether a patient has the resources to manage their care. For example, if a diabetic patient has low income and limited healthcare resources, along with limited access to grocery stores with healthy food choices, their ability to manage their condition can be problematic. They may not be able to afford enough glucose monitoring strips to check their blood glucose as prescribed causing them to only randomly check their glucose levels. They may only have access to a convenience store that does not sell fresh fruits and vegetables.

Essential Facts

The five categories of social determinants of health are economic stability, education, social and community context, health and healthcare, and neighborhood and built environment (Department of Health and Human Services, 2020).

The neighborhood also plays a significant role in health. If the neighborhood is unsafe for the patient to walk and obtain exercise, the patient may be afraid to go out of doors. An unsafe neighborhood may also contribute to psychosocial problems that lead to feelings of loneliness and isolation, which may contribute to complications of certain conditions. Transportation is another concern; if patients do not have available transportation, they may not be able to make their healthcare appointments. When assessing the needs of the patient, all of these factors need to be asked and addressed to ensure that patient-centered care is really being accomplished.

Coaching, phone calls, and online self-management programs ensure that the patient understands follow-up care. Also, making the postdischarge follow-up appointment for the patient is helpful in ensuring that the patient understands they need to follow up with their provider. Be sure to inquire regarding transportation, as this can be a concern for many patients. If transportation is an issue, consulting social work is often helpful in determining transportation alternatives. Aspects of patient-centered care involve interdisciplinary teams that can bridge the gaps in areas of care that nursing is unable to maintain.

Medication Management

Medication reconciliation is one of the leading problems when transitioning patients from or to an acute care facility. Sponsler, Neal, and Kripalani (2015) state that up to "70% of hospitalized discharges involve medication discrepancies ... 50% of patients have a clinically important medication error ... and 20% experience an adverse event" (Katz, 2020, p. 352). These authors also acknowledge that the greater the number of medications a patient is prescribed, the higher the risk for discrepancies to occur. Inadequate communication is the leading factor related to patient mismanagement of medications, but ineffective processes also play a role in this problem.

Inadequate history taking and reconciliation of medication at admission, during admission, and at discharge leads to an incomplete listing of the patient's medications. It is important to reconcile medications at these periods in the patient transition as patient conditions often change, resulting in medications to be discontinued, as well as added to a patient's treatment plan. The Institute for Healthcare Improvement (IHI) (2011) suggests that a team approach should be used when reconciling medications. The team should involve the physician, nurse, and pharmacist to ensure that all medications are listed and have been reviewed with the patient. Sponsler et al. (2015) state that reconciliation processes that include pharmacists have been shown to improve overall outcomes related to medication processes. The initial step in the reconciliation process includes interviewing the patient or family member; if the family is unavailable, contact the PCP for a complete listing of medications. It is always good to obtain a list from the PCP even if the patient and family are present to compare with the patient's list as a means of determining discrepancies and patient adherence to their treatment plan.

When reviewing the medication list, it is best to use communication strategies that would improve gathering of important information. As stated previously under the Communication section, begin with open-ended questions. This might include phrases such as "Tell me what medications you take," "What is the reason you take this medication?" "Are there any over-the-counter medications you take?" "Do you have medications you take that are weekly, monthly, skin patches, or injections?"

Other reconciliation processes include clarifying the dosages and determining how often the patient takes the medication. Nurses must ensure that the dosage is within normal ranges, and if it is not, inquire why the patient is taking a particular dose. Never assume the information the patient has is accurate, and always double-check with other providers if possible. Note if the patient is adhering to the medication regimen, and if not, delve into why the patient may not be. Patients prescribed a weekly medication may forget to take the medication regularly, and it may be helpful to provide the patient with techniques to remind them. Some drugs include specific instructions for the patient to follow when taking the drugs; therefore, emphasizing these requirements is always important. An example of both of these concerns is alendronate sodium for osteoporosis. This drug is taken weekly with specific instructions to take prior to breakfast and remain upright for 20 minutes to avoid esophagitis and related complications. It is important that the patient understands specific instructions, and the rationale behind the instructions, to avoid complications and improve adherence.

When reconciling medications, it is important to critically think about why the patient may be taking the prescribed drugs. Look for medications that may be similar or have the same classification and inquire as to the rationale for taking more than one of these medications. There are times when a patient is administered a formulary medication in the acute care setting and it is then added to the patient's discharge medications along with the previous home medication. Sponsler et al. (2015) state this situation commonly occurs with "statins, antihypertensives, urinary spasmodics and proton pump inhibitors" (p. 356).

If the indication for the medication is lacking, double-check with the patient, the hospitalist, and the PCP to ensure the patient should be taking it. There have been times when patients are prescribed proton pump inhibitors during a hospital stay prophylactically for hospital-induced stress ulcers, and the medication is included in the discharge medication list unnecessarily (Sponsler et al., 2015). When discharging a patient, make sure that the physician does indeed intend for the patient to continue this medication at home. There have also been times during the admission medication reconciliation when the nurse is alerted to conditions that may not be listed in the history. For example, a patient was admitted with amiodarone on their medication list, but there was nothing in the patient's medical record indicating their health history would require this medication. It turned out the patient had a history of atrial fibrillation and was obtaining the medication prescription from a cardiologist instead of the admitting PCP. Omitting a drug such as amiodarone could have been a potentially serious omission if the nurse had not reconciled the medications thoroughly.

When discharging patients, always determine if the patient is able to afford the medication, has access to a pharmacy, and has the ability to obtain their medications from the pharmacy. Make sure they understand the need to follow up with their PCP for refills and any other questions they may have regarding their medications. For patients on multiple medications, some pharmacies offer pill packs that provide the patient's pills in one particular daily or dose package, making it easier for the patient to remember what they are to take and when. The use of medication boxes and medication tool kits can also be helpful to patients in remembering to take their medications. As the coordinator of care, the CNL must delve into all of the needs of the patient when it comes to medication reconciliation to enhance compliance and reduce complications.

INTERDISCIPLINARY TEAM MANAGEMENT

The AACN (2013) states that a fundamental role of the CNL is "team management and collaboration with other health professional team members" (p. 36). The CNL is also to recognize and address risk. There is no place in the daily work of the CNL that these two skills are more important than in the transition of patients from one setting of care to another. The potential risk associated with omissions and communication errors is always great during the transition process. The CNL must use their team management skills in collaborating, communicating, and guiding the interdisciplinary team in determining the best actions to take for each individual patient. This includes ensuring that the plan of care is appropriately and accurately communicated between units, facilities, and care providers.

The CNL must use leadership skills and techniques learned in their programs to lead teams in ensuring each patient is provided the patient-centered care they deserve. Every discipline should be considered when determining who to include in the team to address each individualized need of the patient. Utilizing these skills will prove the value of the CNL professional in enhancing the coordination and transition of patients in any care setting. Scott et al. (2017) eloquently state the rationale for the efforts that the CNL takes in this area of care by saying, "Disease isn't what brings the patient back to the hospital, what brings them back is inability to see their doctor, inability to get food, inability to get their meds" (p. 43).

Clinical Nurse Leader Vignette 7.1: Coordination of Care on a Medical Unit

The CNL on a medical unit was called upon by a registered nurse to intervene for a patient who was very upset regarding a delay in an MRI and lumbar puncture (LP) procedure to determine if surgery was indicated for their condition. The patient had been told by the provider they were to have the procedures done that day. After going and calming the patient, the CNL called the MRI department to see where the patient was on the list. She was informed that the patient was currently not on the daily list as the patient was listed as a "routine" status. This status meant that there was no hurry for the test to be performed. The CNL then called the fluoroscopy department to see when the LP was scheduled. The CNL was informed that the department could not perform the LP as the patient had Plavix on their medical record and that the patient would need to have the Plavix held for 7 days prior to the procedure. The CNL called the patient's wife to verify the last dose of Plavix as the patient was a poor historian. It was determined that the patient would need to wait an additional 5 days before an LP could be done. The CNL notified the physician of the issue who in turn updated the MRI status to stat. The patient received the MRI that day. The results indicated that the LP was not warranted, thus cancelling that procedure. The surgery was then scheduled for the following day. The coordination of care provided by the CNL decreased the patient's anxiety, eliminated the pain and potential complications of an unwarranted invasive procedure, and expedited a surgical procedure, which would potentially reduce the hospitalization time for this patient.

References

American Association of Colleges of Nursing. (2013). *Competencies and curricular expectations for clinical nurse leader education and practice*. Retrieved from https://www.aacnnursing.org/Portals/42/AcademicNursing/CurriculumGuidelines/CNL-Competencies-October-2013.pdf

American Nurses Association. (2012). *The value of nursing care coordination. A white paper of the American Nurses Association* [White Paper]. Retrieved from https://www.nursingworld.org/~4afc0d/globalassets/practiceandpolicy/health-policy/care-coordination-white-paper-3.pdf

Benjamin, R. M. (2010). Improving health by improving health literacy. *Public Health Reports, 125*(6), 784–785. doi:10.1177/003335491012500602

Brooks, A., & John, L. (2018). The surprising power of questions. *Harvard Business Review, 18*(5), 60–67. Retrieved from https://hbr.org/2018/05/the-surprising-power-of-questions

Bucknall, T. K., Hutchinson, A. M., Botti, M., McTier, L., Rawson, H., Hewitt, N. A., ... Chaboyer, W. (2016). Engaging patents and families in communication across transitions of care: An integrative review protocol. *Journal of Advance Nursing, 72*(7), 1689–1700. doi:10.1111/jan.12953

Centers for Medicare and Medicaid Services. (2018). *CMS announces new payment model to improve quality, coordination, and cost-effectiveness for both inpatient and outpatient care.* Retrieved from https://www.cms.gov/newsroom/press-releases/cms-announces-new-payment-model-improve-quality-coordination-and-cost-effectiveness-both-inpatient

The Chronic Care Model. (2019). http://www.improvingchroniccare.org/index.php?p=The_Chronic_CareModel&s=2

Cloonan, P., Wood, J., & Riley, J. B. (2013). Reducing 30-day readmissions health literacy strategies. *The Journal of Nursing Administration, 43*(7/8), 382–387. doi:10.1097/NNA.0b013e31829d6082

Enderlin, C. A., McLeskey, N., Rooker, J. L., Steinhauser, C., D'Avolio, D., Gusewelle, R., & Ennen, K. A. (2013). Review of current conceptual models and frameworks to guide transitions of care in older adults. *Geriatric Nursing, 34,* 47–52. doi:10.1016/j.gerinurse.2012.08.003

Greene, S. M., Tuzzio, L., & Cherkin, D. (2012). A framework for making patient-centered care front and center. *The Permanente Journal, 16*(3), 49–53.

Institute for Healthcare Improvement. (2011). *How-to guide: Prevent adverse drug events by implementing medication reconciliation.* Retrieved from http://www.ihi.org/resources/Pages/Tools/HowtoGuidePreventAdverse-DrugEvents.aspx

Institute of Medicine. (2001). *Crossing the quality chasm. A new health system for the 21st century.* Washington, DC: The National Academies Press.

Katz, B. (2020). *Connecting care for patients.* Burlington: MA: Jones and Bartlett Learning.

Kerstenetzky, L., Birschbach, M. J., Beach, K. F., Hager, D. R., & Kennelty, K. A. (2017). Improving medication information transfer between hospitals, skilled-nursing facilities, and long-term-care pharmacies for hospital discharge transitions of care: A targeted needs assessment using the Intervention Mapping framework. *Research in Social and Administrative Pharmacy, 14,* 138–145. doi:10.1016/.sapharm.2016.12.013

Lamb, G. (2013). *Care coordination: The game changer. How nursing is revolutionizing quality care.* Silver Spring, MD: American Nurses Association.

Lamb, G., & Newhouse, R. (2018). *Care coordination. A blueprint for action for RNs.* Silver Spring, MD: American Nurses Association.

McDonald, K. M., Schultz, E., Albin, L., Pineda, N., Lonhart, J., Sundaram, V., ... Davies, S. (2014). *Care coordination measures atlas (14-0037-EF).* Retrieved from Agency for Healthcare Research and Quality: https://www.ahrq.gov/professionals/prevention-chronic-care/improve/coordination/atlas2014/index.html

National Quality Forum. (2014). *NQF-endorsed measures for care coordination: Phase 3, 2014* [Technical Report]. Retrieved from http://www.qualityforum.org/Publications/2014/12/NQF-Endorsed_Measures_for_Care_Coordination__Phase_3.aspx

Rattray, N. A., Sico, J. J., Cox, L. M., Russ, A. L., Matthias, M. S., & Frankel, R. M. (2017). Crossing the communication chasm: Challenges and opportunities in transitions of care from the hospital to the primary care clinic. *The Joint Commission on Quality and Patient Safety, 43,* 127–137. doi:10.1016/jcjq.2016.11.007

Scott, A. M., Oyewole-Eltu, S., Nguyen, H. Q., Gass, B., Hirschman, K. B., Mitchell, S., ... Williams, M. V. (2017). Understanding facilitators and barriers to care transitions: Insights from project ACHIEVE site visits. *The Joint Commission on Quality and Patient Safety, 43*, 433–447. doi:10.1016/j.jcjq.2017.02.012

Sheikh, F., Gathecha, E., Bellantoni, M., Christmas, C., Lafreniere, J. P., & Arbaje, A. I. (2018). A call to bridge across silos during care transitions. *The Joint Commission on Quality and Patient Safety, 44*, 270–278. doi:10.1016/j/jcjq.2017.10.006

Sponsler, K. C., Neal, E. B., & Kripalani, S. (2015). Improving medication safety during hospital-based transitions of care. *Cleveland Clinic Journal of Medicine, 82*(6), 351–360. doi:10.3949/ccjm.82a.14025

U.S. Department of Health and Human Services. (2020, March 27). *Social determinants of health.* Retrieved from https://www.healthypeople.gov/2020/topics-objectives/topic/social-determinants-of-health

8

Effective Change Management

Ann Deerhake

"It is not the strongest of the species that survive, nor the most intelligent, but the one most responsive to change."
~Charles Darwin

INTRODUCTION

In 21st-century healthcare, change is certainly the rule and not the exception. This frequent occurrence of healthcare change, however, does not mean that change is quick, easy, or consistently well done. Quite the contrary, there is an art and science to implementing positive, lasting culture transformation within healthcare organizations. When honing the art of change, perhaps most important is to consider your ability to influence others as the clinical nurse leader (CNL) within your microsystem. Assessing your personal inventory of change skills is a great place to begin, subsequently moving toward both effective change communication and barrier reduction. Additionally, the science of change is grounded in theory, with multiple change theories available to guide transformation efforts. Another part of your role as a CNL is to carefully choose a theory-based framework on which to identify a need for and construct an effective change management plan. Taking the time to find a theory that fits well with your microsystem is a critical step in the change process. Your role, as a catalyst for change, is to not only build the road toward culture transformation but anticipate and remove obstacles along the way.

After reading this chapter, you will be able to:

1. Reflect upon personal readiness for change
2. Recognize organizational and microsystem barriers to change
3. Describe change communication strategies
4. Develop an evidence-based change implementation and sustainability plan

THE NEED FOR CHANGE IN HEALTHCARE

According to Salmond and Echevarria (2017), healthcare is in crisis because of soaring costs, decreasing quality, and varying needs of an aging, chronically ill population. They continue making a clear statement that nurses and change are partners in healthcare reform: "Nurses are positioned to contribute to and lead the transformative changes that are occurring in healthcare by being a fully contributing member of the interprofessional team" (p. 12). Driven by critical need, and for the first time in nursing, a master's prepared role has been designed specifically to effect change. In the United States, one of every five federal dollars is spent on healthcare, yet the quality of care continues to be subpar (Salmond & Echevarria, 2017). Providing care for aging Americans with multiple chronic illnesses continues to push the system to its limits. This has become a massive economic health problem, affecting all U.S. citizens and the global healthcare market beyond, making it difficult to even imagine what can be done to repair such an incredibly broken system.

On an organizational level, Schein (2017) posits, "A desire for change, for doing something differently, for learning something new, *always begins with some kind of pain or dissatisfaction*" (loc. 6344). As nurses, we know how to assess for pain and dissatisfaction on a patient level, but where do we begin when uncovering multifactorial organizational healthcare issues and leading subsequent change efforts? The concept of disconfirmation, suggested by Schein (2017), is the identification of problem processes or unmet goals within an organization. These disconfirming issues may be long-standing problems that no one has chosen to tackle. CNLs can recognize disconfirmation within organizations by starting at the microsystem level. In fact, you have likely already found problem processes or unmet goals after completing your microsystem assessment (see Chapter 4, Microsystem Assessment and the 5Ps), such as increased pressure ulcer or nurse turnover rates.

Although problems may be identified, that does not mean others in your microsystem will feel they need to be rectified, because many times people rationalize why something is the way it is. When discussing change, surely you have heard others say, "But ... we've always done it THIS way!" The next step is to determine the relationship between staff motivation to fix the problem and trepidation about learning something new. Schein (2017) suggests that survival anxiety happens when people feel they need to make a change because there is a great need, thereby motivating change, whereas learning anxiety occurs when people are afraid they will lose their current status at work if they alter their behavior by learning something new, thus discouraging change. The goal here is not necessarily to increase survival anxiety, but to decrease learning anxiety by recognizing and addressing staff learning concerns (Schein, 2017). In other words, the best way to motivate your microsystem is by making others feel comfortable with how change learning will affect their current role.

Essential Facts

"In 2014, 14.5% (46.3 million) of the U.S. population was age 65 or older and is projected to reach 23.5% (98 million) by 2060. Aging adults experience higher risk of chronic disease" (Office of Disease Prevention and Health Promotion, 2019).

Examining these problems at the microsystem level, both from a specific issue viewpoint and from a synergistic perspective, is a reasonable place to start when considering initiation of change. CNLs are strategically placed at the point of care, facilitating their immersion into the role of change agent within their particular microsystem. Additionally, the generalist nature of the CNL preparation and role enables performance of unbiased assessments of all population and professional issues within a microsystem. This ability to examine all patient and staff factors equally is a prime example of why CNLs do not specialize. First, however, the CNL must assess his or her willingness and aptitude to be the change leader; are you ready?

READYING YOURSELF FOR CHANGE LEADERSHIP

Nurses are leaders, regardless of the role they perform. The nature of the profession gives us countless opportunities to lead at both the point of care and the meeting room. As a CNL, this may be your first experience in officially leading others; however, the likelihood is that you have led for years in different capacities. Whether you have been a primary care nurse, bedside nurse, charge nurse, preceptor, or any other of the countless nursing positions available, you have led from where you are. Nurse leader Linnette Johnson (2017) states, "Leaders must have the moral courage to explore their own leadership attributes, values, and competencies; they must master themselves before they move on to lead others" (p. 160). While reflecting back on past nursing experiences, the question to ask yourself is, "What successful leadership experiences have I had?" Answering this question starts the process of first making needed changes to your leadership style; only then will you be successful in leading change initiatives within your microsystem.

Healthcare leadership expert Catherine Robinson-Walker (2017) outlines a reflective seven-step plan for becoming self-aware (pp. 156–157) and thereby heightening your capacity to lead during change:

1. *Be honest with yourself.* In what ways has your leadership been effective or not so effective in the past? What kind of feedback were you given as a leader? How might you apply this to your current role? How do truly feel about being a change leader?
2. *Critically consider other's viewpoints.* What is the basis for the comments from others? How do their statements fit within the context of the discussion? Is there truth here?
3. *Become conscious of your attitudes, emotional reactions, and internal conversations.* Consider how you respond to others. Are your attitudes and emotions the first thing they see? How might you change this? Taking the time to intentionally think and respond, along with monitoring and, at times, limiting your inner monologue can make a huge difference.
4. *Create your vision.* What kind of job do you want to have? Are your career plans aligned with the job you possess? How could you alter your vision to make yourself the best fit for your microsystem?
5. *Value your assets.* Understand that others may not notice or appreciate what you do well; they may even feel threatened by your abilities. How might you show others your strengths without making them feel defensive or isolated?

6. *Be kind and patient with yourself.* Do not allow insecurity to take over your inner self-talk. In what ways might you allow yourself to work through your thoughts? This will enable you to identify previous bad habits and work toward making better decisions.
7. *Elicit the support of others.* Learn to trust and listen to others. How might including others in your decision-making work for you? Everyone has something unique to bring to the table!

This reflection plan is a reasonable process all nurse leaders should work through; however, it is most critical when preparing to lead change initiatives. Using a framework for reflection and perhaps writing the answers to the preceding questions in your journal will help you to work toward readiness. The University of Melbourne (2017) suggests using the acronym DIEP when reflecting:

D = Describe the key aspects of the experience.
I = Interpret what the experience meant, how it made you feel and insights learned.
E = Evaluate the ways you benefited from the experience.
P = Plan for how the experience will impact your future behavior.

Times of healthcare change can be wrought with frustration and anxiety; possessing a well-defined personal leadership style can help you lead this process effectively. Selecting a specific change framework is the next step in successful change management.

Essential Facts

"Transformational leaders take people where they need to be, not necessarily where they want to be." ~Karen Drenkard (2014)

CHOOSING A CHANGE THEORY

Out of necessity, healthcare has changed dramatically in recent years, and CNLs are charged with facilitating this progression via microsystem change initiatives. In Table 8.1, Salmond and Echevarria (2017) contrast many of the patterns of change within healthcare over the past 20 years, highlighting that new models of healthcare are moving from a sick model of episodic care to an evidence-based well model of continuous health promotion and disease prevention. The CNL role was specifically designed to lead patients and professionals through these shifting paradigms, advocating for well nursing.

Table 8.1

Shifting Healthcare Paradigms: From the Past to the Future

The Past	The Future
Payment for illness or sick care that is triggered by visits to providers and procedures done	Payment for prevention, care coordination, and care management at the primary care level
Greatest financial award for specialized services	Payment for populations—shared risk for use of specialized services
No accountability for inadequate quality. Quality and quality improvement tasked to a department	Value-based payment asking "How well did patients do?" Quality and quality improvement are prime concerns of every practitioner
Quality measured at the individual level	Quality measured at the individual and aggregate levels
Quality measured for a discrete time period	Quality measured over longer periods
Inconsistent access to care	Same-day appointments, timely access
Disrespect	Respect
Top-down hierarchical command and control. Leadership focused on siloed area of care	Team-based, collaborative care requiring integration of care across the continuum
Nursing not leading or not recognized for their contribution to care	Nurses finding their voice and take an active role in shaping the future of healthcare. Nurses recognized for their value in care coordination
Following orders	Advocating for the patient and the family
Focus on task	Focus on excellence and the patient experience

Source: Salmond, S., & Echevarria, M. (2017). Healthcare transformation and changing roles for nursing. *Orthopedic Nursing, 36*(1), 18. doi:10.1097/NOR.0000000000000308

Choosing the most appropriate theory to guide microsystem change initiatives is critical to their success and sustainability. Mitchell (2013) discusses initiating transformation can be quite difficult, yet applying a specific framework can help others to understand and support the process, resulting in positive outcomes. Although many change theories exist, for the purpose of this book, the three chosen by Mitchell to compare and contrast when specifically applying to change initiatives are discussed, including theories by Lewin, Lippett, and Rogers.

Essential Facts

The hardest part of being a change agent is having the confidence to get started. Using a theory developed by change experts can give you the support you need to move past this roadblock.

Perhaps considered the father of change theory, Kurt Lewin established his three-stage change theory of unfreezing, moving, and refreezing. Within the unfreezing stage, change has been identified as necessary. The moving stage constitutes the period of time when change is actually implemented. The final stage in Lewin's process includes refreezing or allowing this change to become the new normal (Mitchell, 2013). Lewin's theory provides a great starting point for microsystem change, yet it is relatively general and does not provide a specific framework of activities. Figure 8.1 shows an enhanced Lewin's Three-Stage Change Model with some realistic steps included, giving you an idea of how you might apply this model to practice.

Everett Rogers continued the evolution of change theory, producing his five-phase approach to change known as the diffusion of innovation theory. The five stages that comprise this theory include (a) knowledge or awareness; (b) persuasion or interest; (c) decision or evaluation; (d) implementation or trial; and (e) confirmation or adoption (see Figure 8.2). Kaminski (2011) suggests that this model focuses on tailoring the planned change to the understanding of those who may adopt the innovation. In other words, as the change agent, you will present this change in different ways to different groups. The innovators, or those who usually embrace technology within your microsystem, will adapt to the change quickly and are

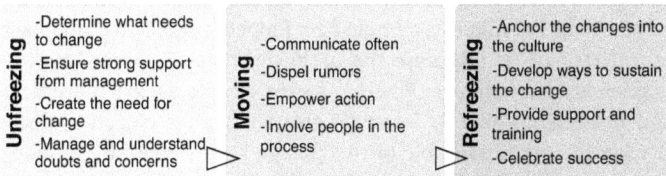

Figure 8.1 Lewin's Three-Stage Change Model with practical applications.
Source: Data from Mitchell, G. (2013). Selecting the best theory to implement planned change. *Nursing Management - UK, 20*(1), 32–37. Retrieved from http://home.nwciowa.edu/publicdownload/Nursing%20Department%5CNUR310%5CSelecting%20the%20Best%20Theory%20to%20Implement%20Planned%20Change.pdf

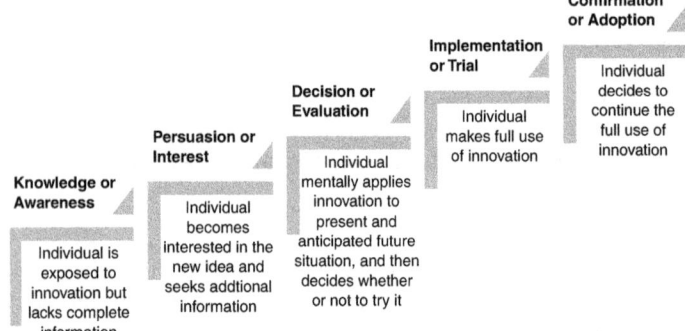

Figure 8.2 Rogers's five-stage diffusion of innovation theory.

Source: Data from Kaminski, J. (2011, June). Diffusion of innovation theory: Theory in Nursing Informatics Column. *Canadian Journal of Nursing Informatics, 6*(2). Retrieved from https://cjni.net/journal/?p=1444

great champions to promote your change project. Early adopters, or those who are leaders within your unit, are likely the group who will be the first to try the change you suggest. The early majority, or those who require rationale for all they do, will need simple yet thorough education before they adopt the innovation. The late majority, or those who are hesitant to respond to any change unless there is a great need, will look to a single leader for guidance. The laggards, or those who are hesitant when it comes to technology and change, are the most difficult to engage. In order to present the innovation plan to your microsystem, all of these groups will need to be identified so that they can receive customized information. Maintaining communication is key with this model (Kaminski, 2011).

Ronald Lippett included terms nurses should be familiar with in his proposed theory. According to Mitchell (2013), he provides a change framework that most nurses can identify with, making it a great choice for microsystem change. Lippett's seven-step approach includes Phase 1. Diagnose the problem; Phase 2. Assess motivation/capacity for change; Phase 3. Assess change agent's motivation and resources; Phase 4. Select progressive change objective; Phase 5. Choose appropriate role of the change agent; Phase 6. Maintain change; and Phase 7. Terminate the helping relationship. After assessing your microsystem and determining your problem, Lippett's change theory provides a step-by-step plan for implementing change (Figure 8.3).

So how do you choose which framework to apply within your microsystem? Do you only choose one theory to guide your change

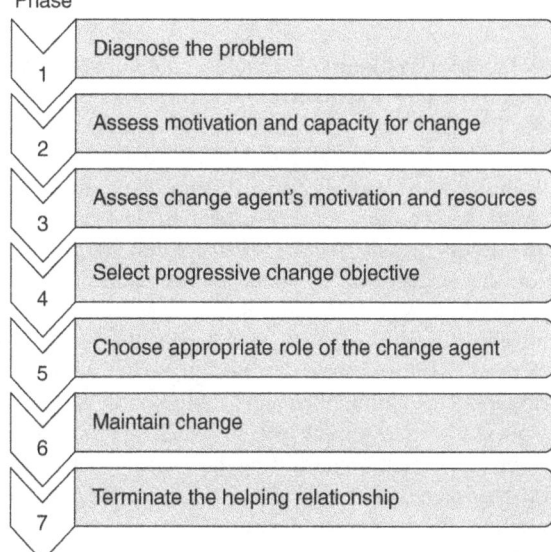

Figure 8.3 Lippett's change theory.

Source: Data from Mitchell, G. (2013). Selecting the best theory to implement planned change. *Nursing Management - UK, 20*(1), 32–37. Retrieved from http://home.nwciowa.edu/publicdownload/Nursing%20Department%5CNUR310%5CSelecting%20the%20Best%20Theory%20to%20Implement%20Planned%20Change.pdf

efforts? The answer here lies within your knowledge of your microsystem. Select a theory based upon what makes the most sense to you. Do not be afraid to personalize your theory framework by combining parts of each theory into your individualized plan. What are the specific issues within your microsystem? Whereas all three theories provide a reasonable approach to change, Roger's theory identifies the differences in the professionals making the change, Lippett's theory discusses the role of the change agent specifically, and Lewin's practical application model highlights barriers to change. Mitchell (2013) suggests how these three theories can work together, providing you with a worksheet to help select the theory, or portions of theory, that work best for you. Also, if one of these does not work for you, find another; there are plenty of other change theories available to you. Then, take your theory selection, place each step in its own page within a "Change" spreadsheet, and start creating your transformation plan!

IDENTIFYING BARRIERS TO CHANGE

Although the theories discussed previously did not specifically discuss barriers, the idea was inferred, aligning with the unfreezing portion of Lewin's theory, the awareness and interest portions of Roger's theory, and phases 1 to 3 of Lippett's theory. Many people, especially protocol-driven healthcare workers, fear change, as it takes them beyond their comfort zone. Mitchell (2013) posits that barriers to change success include the lack of structured framework, finalized action plan, engaged staff, established communication, and supportive leadership. Within the unfreezing stage of Lewin's theory, obtaining administrative support for change and dealing with staff hesitations and anxieties are barriers needing to be addressed before and during implementation of change. Additionally, your microsystem may possess barriers unique to itself, which may be found during microsystem assessment. Determining the barriers to change is vital; the best change plan in the world will not be successful if barriers are not removed or, at minimum, reduced.

Perhaps focusing on two common barriers might be a good place to start. First, do you have administrative support, which is support beyond your microsystem, for your change plan? Although you are planning to implement change within your microsystem only, does your innovation align with the strategic vision of your organization? If not, is there a way to make that happen? Developing a presentation and/or attending organizational meetings to propose and explain your change idea may be necessary. Second, how have those within your microsystem responded thus far? Have you reached out to both managerial and bedside leaders with your general change idea? Is the change you are considering an issue most are concerned about? What effect might the change have on the microsystem's workflow? After considering the answers to these questions, you can begin to categorize the barriers you will need to breakdown, determine workable solutions, and add them to your change spreadsheet within the most appropriate step. There are no easy answers when it comes to removing barriers, but a reasonable strategy includes improving communication among the healthcare team.

COMMUNICATING THE NEED FOR CHANGE

Now that you are working on a plan for decreasing barriers to change, make sure to avoid creating new roadblocks with lack of open and honest communication regarding upcoming and current transformation activities. Interprofessional communication is most important during times of change. While working toward a nursing delivery model that encouraged the best use of each professional's skills, Denney (2019) realized in order to engage staff to take part in the change initiative, they must understand the rationale for the change. Additionally, stakeholders should receive continuous communication about activities throughout the entire transformation process, beginning to end. Similarly, when dealing with the dynamic change that healthcare mergers can bring, Enos (2019) suggests "a major planned event such as an organizational merger requires close communication of intentions with staff, even before all the answers are known" (p. 1). Therefore, designing a communication plan is just as important as developing a financial plan or preparing a timeline for your change project.

When constructing an effective change communication plan, most important may be what you *don't* do:

- *Don't wait until you know every piece of information regarding your change initiative to communicate the plan to others* (Enos, 2019). Some information is better than no information, but be sure let staff know more information is to come and follow up as soon as you can clarify.
- *Don't use the gossip channels to receive or send change information through your microsystem.* Schifalacqua, Costello, and Denman (2009) caution to always consider how information travels within your microsystem, with the "grapevine" being a powerful source of less than accurate information. That being said, many times there may be a grain of truth within the grapevine that needs to be investigated further.
- *Don't allow change communication to only happen randomly.* Mackinson et al. (2018) encourage change agents to schedule in-person conversations, such as presentations in microsystem meetings or small group discussions, as the primary mode of communication. Then supplement with other types of interaction to follow up with staff, such as emails, newsletters, posters, and flyers. Use champions for your change
- *Don't be boring.* Use creativity to draw others in. The typical informational memo in the bathroom is less than original. Is there a new app everyone is talking about that could be used? What about starting "The Story" of your microsystem transformation on a poster in the breakroom and asking for others to continue with their personal change vision? Could you schedule a kickoff event with your microsystem staff to start discussion of upcoming change?

The way you choose to design your communication plan is strictly up to you and your microsystem staff. Many times, telling stories that focus on the reason for the change and how it impacts the patients, healthcare workers, and the organization as a whole can be very effective. It also reveals you, the CNL change agent, as a compassionate, yet influential force in microsystem innovation. The key to change success lies within creating a specific communication process that extends to everyone involved.

Essential Facts

Commitment is contagious. The importance of talking the talk and walking the walk is fundamental to achieving commitment to a project of any magnitude (Schifalacqua, Costello, & Denman, 2009).

IMPLEMENTING THE CHANGE PROCESS

According to Schifalacqua, Costello, and Denman (2009), if nurse leaders want frontline staff to become involved and engaged in change initiatives, the leaders themselves must clearly show their level of commitment to the change. CNLs can do this by becoming fully prepared before implementing a change initiative. All too often, nursing unit leaders prematurely roll out changes before the change structure has been fully developed. Sometimes this happens out of need for a quick response to an adverse event, whereas other instances occur because of lack of knowledge regarding the change process. As a CNL, you can rectify both of these situations by being the point-of-care leader who is readily available to assess the need for change promptly, as well as design and implement a complete change initiative.

Making sure that all components of the change initiative are in place corresponds with the moving portion of Lewin's theory, the evaluation and trial portions of Roger's theory, and phases 4 to 6 of Lippett's theory. Schifalacqua, Costello, and Denman (2009) take this one step further by identifying specific components that should comprise an effective change project, including the following:

- *Charter.* A charter is a document that "explains the purpose, goals and objectives, scope, strategy of approach, key stakeholders, roles and responsibilities, and other important details of the project" (Schifalacqua, Costello, & Denman, 2009, p. 28). Don't let this part overwhelm you! There are templates available that make developing a charter much easier. Taking the time to complete this step helps you define your project as a whole, becoming a great resource for you. Many times, the components given here are included in the charter.

- *Budget.* What monetary resources will you need to complete this change project? The goal here is that "All capital and operating expenses should be included so the true financial impact of the project is clear" (Schifalacqua, Costello, & Denman, 2009, p. 28). Don't hesitate to contact colleagues who work with budgets and other financial planning within your organization for help.
- *Implementation timeline.* What needs to be done and when? This is basically a schedule consisting of all the tasks that need to be completed for your project. "The key to creating effective project plans is to remember that a plan is an approximation of real-life events, not an exact replica" (Schifalacqua, Costello, & Denman, 2009, p. 28). A general rule of thumb is scheduling tasks that take longer than a day but less than 3 weeks should result in a reasonable timeline.
- *Tools.* Are there specific tools you will need to complete this project, technological or otherwise? Do you need items you have no control over, such as Internet connections, in-place policies, or specific data? Completing an inventory of what is needed and where to obtain each item is critical to your success. It is common for projects to be delayed because of lack of specific tools required. Also, checking to see if project management software is available within your organization may be worth the effort.
- *Communication plan.* What methods will you use to keep team members in the communication loop? As discussed previously, defining a specific communication plan is integral to the success of any project, but especially in anxiety-producing change initiatives. This is where CNLs can make a huge difference; including others in change communication invites to become a valued part of the team, fostering innovation ownership.

You can successfully begin implementation only when all of these components of your change initiative are completed. Many times, pressures from administrative, managerial, and frontline staff to make change quickly can push you to begin before your process is actually ready. This is where having patience and being master's-prepared really pays off. You, as the CNL, can role-model your leadership expertise here by staying the course.

> **Essential Facts**
>
> The CDC provides a free charter template at https://www2a.cdc.gov/cdcup/library/templates/CDC_UP_Project_Charter_Template.doc.

SUSTAINING CHANGE

Maintaining change may be the most difficult part of effective change management. In fact, according to Silver et al. (2016), "Unfortunately, up to 70% of organizational change is not sustained" (p. 916). It certainly makes no sense to spend time and money on a change that will not stick. You may think your work is done, but truly, it is just beginning. It is human nature to rest on the laurels of a successful change initiative, especially when there are a bevy of new initiatives needing your attention. However, keeping change intact within your microsystem will require continuous cues from the CNL. One of the components of the practical application of Lewin's refreezing stage includes making the change part of the culture (Mitchell, 2013). How can you embed your change into the culture of your microsystem?

Schein (2017) posits there are six strategies that can be used to ensure culture change actually transpires and is sustained, all of which are related to leader behaviors. How does your microsystem staff perceive your actions? Is it possible to send a clear change message with your personal behavior? Combining both Schein's perspective (2017) and the clinical viewpoint, a CNL should be:

- *Consistent.* Show others what you feel to be important by consistently sending the same message regarding the change. Whether you are at the bedside, in the cafeteria, or in a meeting room, either paying attention to or avoiding a certain issue reveals your priorities to others. Additionally, holding others accountable to maintain change by using champions who also send a consistent message can be very effective (Mount & Anderson, 2015).
- *Calm and caring in crisis.* Unexpected events are part of any business and may happen more often during times of change. Allowing others to see a leader who is concerned for both microsystem staff and the organization as a whole during difficult times will help maintain the culture. Crisis creates anxiety; showing others how to reduce anxiety by remaining calm and

collaborative is a skill that they can take with them wherever they go.
- *Considerate with new change initiatives.* Determining what your microsystem is able to handle, both financially and emotionally, in terms of change is important to consider before planning the next initiative. Critically thinking and talking with others regarding what comes next is key.
- A *point-of-care coach.* You can send emails, write on huddle boards, and post memos in the breakroom, but none of these are as effective as working alongside your microsystem colleagues. The goal is to be intentional yet informal. Putting yourself out there for others to see and hear can inspire them to role-model your behavior, encouraging all staff to maintain the change.
- *Clear when celebrating or commiserating.* As a leader, you will need to give credit when it is due, as well as work toward solutions with staff when things do not go quite as well. Being a good self-monitor in an effort to make sure others are treated equally is extremely important. The need for consistent leadership behavior to maintain change culture cannot be overstated.
- *Critical when choosing new colleagues.* When new members are being considered for hire into the microsystem, you have to contemplate if they will work well within the new culture that has been created. While many times we look to current microsystem staff for inspiration, it may be reasonable to reflect upon what new staffing needs may be required because of the change. Locating and employing members with characteristics that support the change is critical.

Although daunting at times, applying all of these components to your CNL role will help you sustain change within your microsystem. It makes sense to work hard to preserve the great work you have done!

Clinical Nurse Leader Vignette 8.1: A Consolidation Near to My Heart

With much emotion, I remember the day when the ICU unit manager told me that we would be combining with the cardiovascular intensive care unit (CVICU) next door. A few years earlier, we had moved the CVICU and open-heart step-down patients to a dedicated unit, very much pleasing the CV surgeons, and now, we were tearing it all apart. This change project was to be done out of staffing necessity, yet everyone was unhappy: ICU nurses, CVICU nurses, step-down nurses, CV surgeons ... the list goes on and on. As the CNL for both units, all I could think about was where do we start to make this change happen with the least amount of screaming and crying?

The ICU unit manager and I decided on a consistent, true message we would send: This consolidation had to be done for patient safety and staff support reasons. We simply had to recover the CVICU patients in the larger ICU unit so enough CVICU-trained nurses were available to help with patients upon return from surgery. The tension and anxiety between the groups of nurses was almost overwhelming. Bringing them together for a meeting was both good and bad in that they were collaborative, but impatient with one another. Developing a calm atmosphere was something we strived for but did not achieve right away. We determined, at that point, this was all of the change these units could handle; no other quality improvement initiatives would be implemented any time soon, although administration had several they were requesting be done.

We did, however, provide education so those nurses changing units would be prepared to care for different types of patients. The ICU nurses were educated regarding open-heart patients, and the CVICU and step-down nurses were educated regarding med–surg, trauma, and neuro patients. Additionally, I was at the bedside helping and coaching as needed and the unit manager made frequent rounds, both of us striking up informal conversations frequently. Slowly, as time passed, the new unit culture was established. Successes were celebrated, and problems addressed. New staff were hired, including the transfer of some of the open-heart step-down staff to ICU. Yes, we created a new culture within the ICU, but no, the memories of what had been will be ever present for many. And perhaps, that's how it should be.

Ann Deerhake, DNP, RN, CNL, CCRN

References

Denney, S. (2019). Driving change from the bottom up in a top-down culture: Disruptive innovation: One organization's "lessons learned" in gaining stakeholder acceptance. *Nurse Leader, 17*(4), 360–364. doi:10.1016/j.mnl.2018.11.004

Drenkard, K. (2014). Change is a matter of perspective. *Nurse Leader, 12*(1), 72. doi:10.1016/j.mnl.2013.12.007

Enos, G. (2019). In planning major organization change, communicate with staff early and often. *Mental Health Weekly, 29*(19), 1–3. doi:10.1002/MHW.31895

Johnson, L. (2017). Sage advice: Leaders change the world. *Nurse Leader, 15*(3): 160–161. doi:10.1016/j.mnl.2017.03.011

Kaminski, J. (2011, June). Diffusion of innovation theory: Theory in Nursing Informatics Column. *Canadian Journal of Nursing Informatics, 6*(2). Retrieved from https://cjni.net/journal/?p=1444

Mackinson, L., Corey, J., Kelly, V., O'Reilly, K., Stevens, J., Desanto-Madeya, S., ... Foley, J. (2018). Nurse project consultant: Critical care nurses move beyond the bedside to affect quality and safety. *Critical Care Nurse, 38*(3), 54–66. doi:10.4037/ccn2018838

Mitchell, G. (2013). Selecting the best theory to implement planned change. *Nursing Management - UK, 20*(1), 32–37. Retrieved from http://home.nwciowa.edu/publicdownload/Nursing%20Department%5CNUR310%5CSelecting%20the%20Best%20Theory%20to%20Implement%20Planned%20Change.pdf

Mount, A., & Anderson, I. (2015). Driving change—not just a walk in the park: The role of the nurse champion in sustained change. *Nurse Leader, 13*(4), 36–38. doi:10.1016/j.mnl.2015.06.003

Office of Disease Prevention and Health Promotion. (2019). *Healthy people 2020, topics & objectives, older adults*. Retrieved from https://www.healthypeople.gov/2020/topics-objectives/topic/older-adults

Robinson-Walker, C. (2017). Coaching forum: Installing self-awareness and lasting change. *Nurse Leader, 15*(3), 156–157. doi:10.1016/j.mnl.2017.03.010

Salmond, S., & Echevarria, M. (2017). Healthcare transformation and changing roles for nursing. *Orthopedic Nursing, 36*(1), 12–25. doi:10.1097/NOR.0000000000000308

Schein, E. (2017). *Organizational culture and leadership* (Kindle ed.). The Jossey-Bass Business & Management Series. Hoboken, NJ: Wiley.

Schifalacqua, M., Costello, C., & Denman, W. (2009). Roadmap for planned change, part 1: Change leadership and project management. *Nurse Leader, 7*(2), 26–52. doi:10.1016/j.mnl.2008.06.001

Silver, S., McQuillan, R., Harel, Z., Weizman, A., Thomas, A., Nesrallah, G., ... Chertow, G. (2016). How to sustain change and support continuous quality improvement. *Clinical Journal of the American Society of Nephrology: CJASN, 11*(5), 916–924. doi:10.2215/CJN.11501015

University of Melbourne. (2017, June 1). *Reflective writing* [Video file]. Retrieved from https://youtu.be/SntBj0FIApw

9

Advocacy for Nursing and Populations

Ann Deerhake

"Unless someone like you cares a whole awful lot, Nothing is going to get better. It's not."

~Dr. Seuss, *The Lorax*

INTRODUCTION

Who is better to advocate for patients and populations than the nursing professionals who arguably spend the most time caring for them? Who is a more reasonable candidate to advocate for the nursing profession as a whole than nurses themselves? The very essence of nursing requires those within the profession to change their way of thinking, advancing from a layperson to an expert when it comes to patient care. While attending college to obtain a nursing degree, "each learner is surrounded by ideas and, in this immersive context, gradually integrates the aspirational ideals, skillsets, values, and knowledge of the profession into a robust and personalized commitment" (Thorne, 2018, p. 2). Regardless of specific nursing healthcare roles, nurses gain daily insight into a multitude of healthcare issues by being present at a variety of venues, including, but certainly not limited to, the patient bedside, exam room, procedure suite, or meeting table. This knowledge needs to be conveyed to our patients, as well as to those who make both organizational policy and governmental regulatory decisions.

Extending practice beyond the nurse–patient care comfort zone can be intimidating for many; however, nurses are experts when it comes to planning and delivering care, empowering them to be proficient healthcare advocates. While state nurse practice acts throughout the country oblige all nurses to be advocates, clinical nurse leaders (CNLs) have been particularly groomed for this role, via master's education. The American Association of Colleges of Nursing (AACN; 2013) lists "Advocacy for patients, communities, and the health professional team" as an essential CNL practice component (p. 5). The foundation of the CNL role was built on healthcare advocacy.

After reading this chapter, you will be able to:

1. Differentiate advocacy activities within patient, organizational, and policy levels of care
2. Identify the role of the nurse and the CNL in professional nursing advocacy
3. Reflect upon your ability to be a both a patient and nursing profession advocate

PATIENT ADVOCACY

Essential Facts

"For the 17th year in a row, registered nurses top the list of the most honest and ethical professions according to the latest Gallup poll" (Colduvell-Gaines, 2019, para. 1).

Fragmentation of Care

Patients and families trust nurses to assist them in times of need. Whether it is at the bedside during critical illness, the office during chronic illness, the delivery room during the beginning of life, or the home during end of life, nurses are expected to be there for skill and support, in multiple capacities. In years past, patient care was coordinated by the patient or the family physician; however, now it has become a very difficult, time-consuming nursing role. The increase in specialized healthcare providers, constant changes in technology, and complexity of financial policies have divided care in such a way that navigating the healthcare system successfully has become beyond many patients' capabilities.

As we learned in Chapter 3, Leadership Within a Complex Environment (chaos, complexity, and systems thinking), healthcare is complex by design, existing on the edge of chaos in an effort to create high-performing complex adaptive systems. Within these systems, the greatest challenge is empowering the multiple components to work well on their own and, perhaps more important, work well with each other. This synergy is difficult to achieve, resulting in gaps in care that even the most healthcare savvy consumers have trouble hurdling, as well as creating barriers to accessing care. It is critical to understand that access to care is not simply about geographical logistics, but about the ease of use within the healthcare system. Each member of the healthcare team has a personal, well-intended agenda when it comes to patient care; aligning these is perhaps the most important reason the CNL role was envisioned.

So, what does the CNL actually do to decrease care fragmentation? According to the AACN (2013), CNLs are to laterally integrate patient care while leading the healthcare team in professional collaboration efforts. Fundamentally, CNLs are charged with bringing the healthcare team together to close the gaps in care. Being intentional by employing open lines of communication, finding holes in processes and disseminating information transparently is a critical part of the CNL role. Also, role modeling professionalism in ways that let others know all healthcare team members are important to the microsystem purpose is key; no single person can produce excellent patient outcomes without the support of others. This can be done by obtaining knowledge regarding the specific work of each healthcare team member within your microsystem, along with careful consideration of how ancillary microsystems affect the internal workings of your microsystem. Although this takes time and effort, the result is twofold: Not only will you learn multitudes of information, but you will also establish yourself as an authentic, transformative leader. Only then can you proceed to assist patients in need of navigating this fragmented healthcare system.

Essential Facts

> State nurse practice acts as well as ethical codes from both national and international organizations require nurses to be patient advocates.

Navigation of the Healthcare System

While all nurses are patient advocates, those nurses who work in roles of care coordination and nurse navigation may be the most familiar when it comes to assisting patients through the healthcare system. While these roles have been created in recent decades, the newest role along this vein is that of the CNL. Some CNLs may work in these capacities, yet they have the education to provide so much more to current and future patients. While digging to the root of issues and solving them internally is the best way to repair broken processes, American healthcare has become a system full of external quick fixes. Not only can CNLs assist patients through the healthcare system, but they can solve problems using evidence along the way, enabling the next patient to pass through more quickly and safely. It is important to remember that CNLs work at the microsystem level, helping patients move through their microsystem and on to the next, creating the need for CNLs within every microsystem. The end result is an expert network of professionals specifically and strategically placed to support patients and their families, resulting in more efficient use of the healthcare team and increased patient satisfaction.

One of the best ways to help patients navigate healthcare is to know your microsystem well, which has been discussed in regard to closing healthcare team gaps. The next step is to become knowledgeable about the most common community microsystems your patients may interact with, including hospital units, ancillary departments, outpatient settings, primary care offices, community health clinics, rehabilitation centers, local pharmacies, laboratories, and many others. As the information manager of your microsystem, it is necessary to become well versed in all of this information and create a database resource for both the healthcare team and patients to utilize. While CNLs are masters of finding and disseminating information, working in concert with nurse navigators and care coordinators to create a fluid resource that works for all makes sense. Once again, collaborating with those who know is a valuable skill to hone, as well as a healthcare team satisfier. Additionally, using these resources can also assist patients beyond times of illness by becoming a framework for wellness.

Promoting Wellness

While patients and their families primarily seek out nurses for help in times of illness and in times of watchful wellness such as pregnancy, it is critical that the nursing profession educates them regarding the paradigm shift from treating illness to preserving health. In 1893, Florence Nightingale discussed the concepts of "sick nursing" and "health nursing," positing that these are two very different but necessary areas in which nurses can support patients while they work toward their best state of health (Beck, 2010, p. 318). Although nurses have been advocating for wellness care for many years, in recent decades, caring for oneself in an effort to prevent disease has become a hot topic in healthcare. Murdaugh, Parsons, and Pender (2019) make an insightful statement: "Health can exist without illness, but illness never exists without health as its context" (p. 8). In other words, it is important to consider that individuals may have different definitions of illness, based upon how they perceive the concept of health. For example, a person living without chronic disease may define health as living life without any type of physical or psychological problems, whereas those with chronic disease may define health as living life without pain. When individual health is defined more broadly as actualization of human potential, it has been called wellness (Murdaughet et al., 2019).

Facilitating patient wellness is a common objective for nurses, regardless of the specific nursing role they perform. First, assessing patients for wellness needs such as screenings, support groups, and annual routine care must take place. As clinicians, CNLs possess advanced assessment skills, enabling patient needs within the microsystem to be holistically discovered and addressed. Next, connecting patients with resources such as low-cost preventive care to maintain and improve health is the goal. As a collaborative team member and lateral integrator, CNLs can unite patients with professionals who have the common goal of achieving and maintaining wellness. Lastly, as outcome managers, it is essential that CNLs continually evaluate the needs of those within their microsystem, updating plans of care as necessary. As needs change, the CNL may need to repeat the assess, connect, and evaluate cycle in order to provide individuals with the most current information regarding their health.

Murdaugh et al. (2019) suggest individual health suffers if the society around the individual is unhealthy. Nurses are not restricted to caring for patients in traditional settings and are now present in a variety of new venues, including organizational wellness programs and telehealth offerings. The coaching aspect of wellness combined with technology allows nurses to reach patients where they are within the community. Nurses can work to improve the health of the individual; however, people do not live in a vacuum. Many times, patients are efficacious with self-care within the healthcare setting, but upon returning back to their home, they do a poor job of making health decisions and caring for themselves. Although this occurs for many reasons, certainly the environmental effect is one of the most compelling. The question to ask here is, how is the home environment and surrounding community a positive or negative influence on a patient's health? This illustrates the need for nurse advocacy, specifically CNL advocacy, on levels beyond that of the individual. CNLs can intervene to improve outcomes on several levels, starting with developing effective patient and family education to spearheading community offerings to increase awareness of environmental effects, including social influence, on health. Once again, this requires effort outside of standard nurse work, but truly, it is a responsibility of the CNL role.

PROFESSIONAL NURSING ADVOCACY

According to Thorne (2018, p. 2), humanity's faith in nursing comes "from a strong system of nursing care that becomes a safety net in advance of, during and following a health crisis, a support system for persons who are struggling, and a carative system for those in need." Patients look to nurses for holistic care during times when they are most vulnerable, expecting nurses to be their advocate if the situation arises. However, those in need may not be patients or even families, but other professionals within nursing or interdisciplinary professions. Nursing's support of other healthcare team members results in staff retention and thereby better patient outcomes. In essence, advocating for the healthcare team is also advocating for patients.

Historically, nursing advocacy occurs most frequently at the patient bedside, with the nurse advocating for the patient. CNLs lead at the point of care and can use their advanced education to identify problems requiring leadership support and work toward awareness and amelioration. There are many other settings where professionals with or without healthcare experience could garner insight and guidance from nursing expertise, including healthcare organizations, local communities, state districts, national governments, and global populations. All of these settings allow for nursing advocacy by way of bettering nursing work environments, education, and empowerment, which in turn improves patient outcomes in the long term.

Essential Facts

When working with individuals, CNLs should implement strategies that work toward altering the "knowledge, attitudes, beliefs, practices, and behaviors of Individuals" (Keller, Strohschein, Lia-Hoagberg, & Schaffer, 2004, p. 457).

Within the Microsystem

Working toward nurse empowerment, healthy work environments and great patient outcomes start in the microsystem and build throughout an organization. Advocacy within these smallest functional units is critical to its success. The AACN CNL implementation task force designed the CNL role to be one of advocacy and altruism, requiring CNLs to "advocate(s) for clients, particularly the most vulnerable" and "take(s) risks on behalf of clients and colleagues" (AACN, 2007). CNLs are the clinical experts and team managers within their microsystem, positioning them as knowledgeable advocates for both patients and staff alike. The goal here is to be proactive with advocacy and, in other words, work toward preventing fires from starting instead of putting out fires when they occur. There is a time and place for spontaneous advocacy; however, this should be the exception and not the rule.

In-the-moment advocacy is expected of all nurses, given their place within healthcare. Nurses are the eyes and ears of many practitioners, spending the most time at the patient's bedside; therefore, they likely know the patient's wants and needs better than any other healthcare team member. The important piece here is for nurses to present themselves as professional, rational advocates, whether advocating for patients or staff. While many times passion drives the nurse during spontaneous advocacy, it is critical that nurses provide all of the relevant information necessary for others to make informed patient healthcare or organizational policy decisions.

> **Essential Facts**
>
> "Rationality involves using logic, explanation and information to persuade someone" (Geertshuis, Morrison, & Cooper-Thomas, 2015, p. 231).

Perhaps the most efficient way that CNLs can determine planned advocacy interventions for patients and microsystem staff is by increasing exposure to the system and thereby awareness of its function. Positioning yourself within the innerworkings of your unit will allow you to obtain direct knowledge of problems and possible solutions. A simple five-step sensory process can be used to frame this activity:

1. *Look for leads.* Critically observing others is a necessary first step toward determining the needs of your microsystem. What issues are you seeing in regard to staff and patients? Can you group them into common themes? Are they new or old issues? Do they affect communication?
2. *Listen for lucidity.* Actively listening to others many times occurs simultaneously with observing their behavior; however, when focusing on *only* listening, you may be surprised at what you hear. Does the behavior you observed align with what people are saying? If not, why?
3. *Sniff for significance.* Dig deeper into the data you have uncovered. Are these issues superficial complaints that indicate much deeper issues? Are they small concerns that have been inflated into bigger issues? Who might you talk with to clarify current and discover further information?
4. *Taste for truth.* Analyze the information you have collected. Does this ring true to your experience within the microsystem? Do microsystem leaders preach collaboration, yet you have uncovered poor communication among practitioners? Take time here to consider your position.
5. *Feel for focus.* Reflect upon what you have learned and take action. What is the advocacy goal? Start with a maximum of three interventions that could be implemented to reach this goal, such as increasing issue awareness, providing needed education, and monitoring future practice.

Moving through this framework can help you alleviate doubts, boost your confidence, and allow you to take action within your microsystem. Once you have learned to be an active supporter and rational communicator at this level, you can consider moving to community and organizational advocacy and activism.

Essential Facts

When working with communities, CNLs should implement strategies that address "community norms, community attitudes, community awareness, community practices, and community behaviors" (Keller, Strohschein, Lia-Hoagberg & Schaffer, 2004, p. 455).

Within the Community

Imagine the possibilities for improved health outcomes by simply connecting the healthcare team with patients in their home and community settings. Regardless of the type of healthcare setting in which you provide CNL services, your patients will return to and be constantly influenced by their home environment. Bringing excellent care to populations is becoming more of a reality with expanding nursing roles and constantly evolving technology. CNLs are educated to laterally integrate and coordinate interdisciplinary team expertise at the point of care, making those working in the role prime candidates to develop and advocate for community health programs and initiatives. Strategies that CNLs can use to get involved in community level advocacy are as follows:

1. *Look for leads.* Investigating the disparities in your neighborhood by becoming an active member of the community is an important starting point for determining population needs. Perhaps attending local events, participating as a community board member or even reading the local paper or online social chat can give you clues into what health issues exist in your area. Local government and healthcare websites may provide ideas as well.
2. *Listen for lucidity.* Open your ears everywhere you go, whether it is a restaurant, beauty salon, auto shop, grocery store, school, or any other of the countless common spaces in your community. The questions such as "What health issues are concerning to others?"

and "Are there problems specific to diverse community populations, such as those of differing age, race, religion, socioeconomic status, or sexual orientation?" critically reflect upon these data to compare what you have heard and seen.

3. *Sniff for significance.* Behaviors seen and complaints heard frequently indicate the most common issues within a community. Do these correspond with a particular health problem? Can you recognize disparities that correlate with the health issues you have identified? For example, if you are seeing poorly kept green space in your community and hearing parents complain about child sedentarism, is there a connection? Taking the time now to analyze your data and corroborate your findings with health demographic information will help you prioritize your advocacy efforts.

4. *Taste for truth.* It is critical to contemplate the possibility of community involvement in your advocacy plan. How much work are the residents truly willing to do to improve the area in which they live? Are there community leaders, business owners, and resident volunteers who are willing to contribute time and money to make their neighborhood healthier? Much like leading an interdisciplinary team, working with a diverse group of community members will ensure you have chosen the most pressing health initiative. Bringing healthcare team and community members together by meeting at a local coffee shop or community center to discuss the answers to these questions is one way to get started.

5. *Feel for focus.* Now that you have identified the health issues that plague your community the most, how will you work to alleviate these complex problems? Many times, supporting one community change can affect another. Using your newly formed community team to design appropriate interventions for residents is key. Choosing offerings that will encompass more than one healthcare issue while engaging community members may provide the most value for the community. So, if the community children are sedentary and the adults have a high rate of diabetes, perhaps reworking the green spaces as specific exercise areas for both would be a reasonable plan.

With community advocacy and increased wellness comes healthier populations and reduced chronic illness, potentially resulting in more effective healthcare utilization and increasing access to care for all community members. It is feasible to consider that improving the health of community microsystems will also improve state mesosystems and the national macrosystem, answering many healthcare woes.

Essential Facts

When CNLs advocate at the systems level, the strategy is to influence "organizations, policies, laws, and power structures. The focus is on the systems that impact health, not directly on individuals and communities" (Keller, Strohschein, Lia-Hoagberg & Schaffer, 2004, p. 457).

Within the Organization

While the CNL role is designed to take place within the microsystem, certainly the overarching goal is to improve healthcare in its entirety, one organization at a time. Using microsystem data to educate and strengthen organizational macrosystems is a great CNL strategy to improve the health of organizations. After all, who knows more about the successes and failures of your microsystem better than you? Furthermore, many of you have pondered, "If this initiative works well in my microsystem, I wonder how it would work in other areas of the organization?" Other managers without CNLs in their ranks may have actually sought you out, requesting information on your successes and ideas on how to make change within their areas as well. While some projects, such as ventilator-assisted pneumonia prevention, are only conducted within specific microsystems, others, such as fall prevention, may be needed throughout a facility. CNLs, as systems thinkers and experts within their microsystems, can bring valuable information to decision-makers and connect professionals at the front line to those within administrative offices. This is critical collaboration that needs to take place in order to narrow the healthcare hierarchical gap, as well as bridge the intradisciplinary nursing communication disconnect.

In an effort to achieve excellent patient outcomes, collaboration within organizations needs to occur among all types of professionals. From a CNL perspective, collaborative advocacy depends upon the nursing care delivery system within your facility. Does the larger organization in which your microsystem exists utilize CNLs throughout settings? If so, has a CNL networking structure been created, such as regularly scheduled meetings dedicated to discussing CNL work, including successes and failures? If this is the case, a CNL professional mesosystem has been built, allowing for a united front consisting of likeminded individuals, a powerful tool in advocacy efforts. If not, have you considered advocating for more CNLs within your organization? This would entail advocating for a stronger advocacy structure, not to mention improved professional communication, staff satisfaction, and patient outcomes! In other words, determining the influence of your individual CNL role compared with that of a network of CNLs throughout your organization is an important step in deciding upon how to go about advocacy activities.

While you, as the CNL, are the expert within your microsystem, it is important to remember that you are not a macrosystem authority. Interaction with administrative healthcare business leaders requires CNLs to frame issues based upon an organizational perspective. As both a chief clinical officer and executive nurse fellow, Bonnie Clipper, RN, posits that nurse executives are required to work toward "influencing innovation, spanning boundaries, collaboration, expanding the accessibility and use of technology and, perhaps particularly important, courage" (as cited in Larson, 2017, para. 6). Based on these five components, you will need to hypothesize how a particular microsystem advocacy issue or initiative may affect the macrosystem, including the financial implications. A well-formulated advocacy plan that is innovative, collaborative, technologically sound, and proven to be cost-neutral will likely be successful when presented at the administrative table.

CNLs can become liaisons who connect the front line to the C-suite by using the same sensory process and applying their microsystem expertise to the organizational macrosystem:

1. *Look for leads.* From a CNL perspective, take notice of the actions of those in management and administrative roles. What microsystem initiatives align with overall macrosystem goals? How does the activity within your microsystem support the strategic plan of the organization? Are there education or communication disconnects between your microsystem and the organization?
2. *Listen for lucidity.* Every conversation with upper management is an opportunity to learn more about the operation of the C-suite, as well as educate others regarding your microsystem. Initially, it is important to listen from an impartial perspective, taking your microsystem bias out of the picture. Does the behavior you observed match what you are hearing? Then, add your microsystem back into the picture. How does this conversation affect your microsystem? Do you need to advocate for your microsystem so others understand its particular needs?
3. *Sniff for significance.* Consider the information you have garnered on all levels. Educating yourself regarding the organizational mission, strategic vision and core values will help you determine if a

particular project is significant to administrators. How does your microsystem fit into the larger macrosystem picture? Do your administrators understand that to improve the macrosystem, you must first work at the point of care to create a high-functioning microsystem? In what ways can your microsystem contribute to the improvement activities of the organization? What further information do you need to gather and which stakeholders might be of assistance?

4. *Taste for truth.* Contemplate the value that those macrosystem-focused administrators place on your microsystem. Are they taking your microsystem advocacy seriously? Are your administrators ready to work alongside you to improve your microsystem and thereby the macrosystem? Do they understand the importance of systems theory in organizational quality improvement? If not, imparting more education may be necessary; gaining genuine administrative support for CNL activities is critical to role success and good patient outcomes.

5. *Feel for focus.* Again, reflect upon what you have learned. Take action once you have determined which initiatives align most closely between the micro- and macrosystems. Organize your quality improvement plan by prioritizing which goals are most important to all.

Organizational culture many times dictates advocacy activities. Completing a thorough five-step assessment will likely help you identify those who facilitate or impede advocacy. Putting together an effective, supportive, and synergistic change team is the goal.

Within the Nation and Throughout the World

Nurses are the light of the world. Turale and Kunaviktikul (2019) clearly state "For nurses around the world to take their place at decision-making tables, and to be more fully engaged in policymaking and reform, they need to have the requisite knowledge, skills and attitudes" (p. 303). Nurses leading advocacy activities at state, national, and global levels is heady stuff; how can nurses prepare for this? CNLs specifically have been educated to apply evidence to care, as well as communicate effectively in a variety of ways, providing the critical link in evidence-based healthcare team collaboration. Thus, if CNLs can laterally integrate groups of professionals into evidentiary working teams, certainly this same expertise can also be used throughout governmental advocacy efforts. What might this look like?

1. *Look for leads.* Do you possess a healthcare concern, which invokes passion inside of you? Many nurses do. The list is endless, from new life to end-of-life issues and everything in between, within a multitude of settings and populations. Frequently, but not always, issues nurses feel strongly about are things they have been exposed to personally and/or professionally, leaving them with a certain amount of experiential knowledge regarding the problem. Searching the scholarly literature and reading governmental websites regarding your concerns can help you understand the full scope of your chosen advocacy issue and provide support for your cause.
2. *Listen for lucidity.* When it comes to your issue, what are others saying? Are they credible sources of information? Do they speak supported by knowledge of the issue or based primarily on their personal opinion? Face-to-face, email, and social media interactions can provide venues for communication about your issue. Differentiating between knowledge and opinion, along with comparing and contrasting what you have heard with what you have seen and read in your research, is critical to the success of your advocacy plan.
3. *Sniff for significance.* Is your chosen issue truly what you thought it was? Or has it changed after looking and listening? Can you substantiate the information you have collected by talking with experts or correlating with the literature? A great strategy could include making a list of stakeholders currently affected by the issue, as well as those who may be affected in the future, such as legislators. Conducting interviews with these groups will likely bring forth rich data, which will help you identify exactly what it is you are advocating to initiate or change.
4. *Taste for truth.* Consider your present position on this issue now that you have become fully informed. Is working toward solving this problem worth your time and professional advocacy efforts? If so, be prepared to become a subject matter expert and point person for both laymen and professionals in regard to your issue. Finding others who share similar views to collaborate with may give you confidence as well as divide the advocacy workload.
5. *Feel for focus.* What is the most important change you would like to make in regard to your issue? It is not likely that you will be able to advocate for all components of a complex health problem; narrowing it down to the priority issue is an important step toward advocacy success. Certainly, there will be opportunities to work on other parts of the bigger issue at a later time.

The final step for all levels of advocacy is to position yourself in a place you can be seen and heard. We have come full circle, starting with a passion, developing it into an advocacy issue that can be discussed and now letting others know our thoughts and ideas. Advocacy needs exist throughout all levels of professional nursing practice, from the bedside to global meetings. Where does your issue take you?

> **Clinical Nurse Leader Vignette 9.1:**
> **Florence Nightingale in the 21st Century**
>
> *Imagine what Florence Nightingale could or would have done if she'd had the technology we have today! That is exactly what the cofounders of the Nightingale Initiative for Global Health (NIGH) did. Fax machines, Internet browsers, email accounts, and smart phones are a part of everyday life in the new millennium. By utilizing these and other technologies, this self-organized group of global volunteers has created "The Nightingale Declaration for a Healthy World," an online, participatory doctrine available to nurses and others who are ready to commit to improving the health of our world (NIGH, 2019). This declaration, with more than 25,000 followers from 106 countries, calls nurses to action by promoting the goal of global health. Their plan is to achieve this lofty objective by connecting nurses together on personal, professional, and societal levels.*
>
> *NIGH is working in conjunction with the Charter for Compassion movement to alleviate "pain and suffering in communities," "promote education for all that is based in secular ethics, social emotional learning, kindness, and compassion," and work toward attaining the "17 UN Sustainable Development Goals," including "freeing our world from poverty, hunger and [advocating for] good health and well-being" (Charter for Compassion, 2019). This is nursing advocacy at its finest.*
>
> *The mantra of this advocacy group comprises "DARING to tell the untold and forgotten stories of global health; CARING to engage and empower the public voices of nurses, midwives and concerned citizens; and SHARING this opportunity wherever possible, with everyone—everywhere!" (Beck, Dossey, & Rushton, 2013, p. 367).*
>
> *To learn more, go to https://www.nighvision.net or https://charterforcompassion.org.*

References

American Association of Colleges of Nursing. (2007). *White paper on the education and role of the clinical nurse leader.* Washington, DC: Author.

American Association of Colleges of Nursing. (2013). *Competencies and curricular expectations for the clinical nurse leader in education and practice.* Retrieved from https://www.aacnnursing.org/Portals/42/News/White-Papers/CNL-Competencies-October-2013.pdf

Beck, D. (2010). Expanding our Nightingale horizon: Seven recommendations for 21st-century nursing practice. *Journal of Holistic Nursing, 28*(4), 317–326. doi:10.1177/0898010110387780

Beck, D., Dossey, B., & Rushton, C. (2013). Building the Nightingale initiative for global health—NIGH: Can we engage and empower the public voices of nurses worldwide? *Nursing Science Quarterly, 26*(4), 366–371. doi:10.1177/0894318413500403

Charter for Compassion. (2019). *Join the movement.* Retrieved from https://charterforcompassion.org/

Colduvell-Gaines, K. (2019). *Nurses rank most honest profession 17 years in a row.* Retrieved from https://nurse.org/articles/nursing-ranked-most-honest-profession

Geertshuis, S., Morrison, R., & Cooper-Thomas, H. (2015). It's not what you say, it's the way that you say it: The mediating effect of upward influencing communications on the relationship between leader-member exchange and performance ratings. *International Journal of Business Communication, 52*(2), 228–245. doi:10.1177/ 2329488415572784

Keller, L., Strohschein, S., Lia-Hoagberg, B., & Schaffer, M. (2004). Population-based public health interventions: Practice-based and evidence-supported. Part I. *Public Health Nursing, 21*(5), 453–468. doi:10.1111/J.0737-1209.2004.21509.X

Larson, L. (2017). The rapidly evolving role of nurse execs. *H&HN: Hospitals & Health Networks, 91*(3), 28–31. Retrieved from https://www.hhnmag.com/articles/8029-the-rapidly-evolving-role-of-nurse-executives

Murdaugh, C., Parsons, M., & Pender, N. (2019). *Health promotion in nursing practice* (8th ed., Kindle Locations 661–662, Kindle ed.). New York, NY: Pearson.

Nightingale Initiative for Global Health [NIGH]. (2019). *The Nightingale declaration for a healthy world.* Retrieved from https://www.nighvision.net/nightingale-declaration.html

Thorne, S. (2018). In search of our collective voice. *Nursing Inquiry, 25*, e12266. doi:10.1111/nin.12266

Turale, S., & Kunaviktikul, W. (2019). The contribution of nurses to health policy and advocacy requires leaders to provide training and mentorship. *International Nursing Review, 66*(3), 302–304. doi:10.1111/inr.12550

10

Disseminating Accomplishments

Janice Wilcox

*"Your words will tell others what you think.
Your actions will tell them what you believe."*

~T. D. Jakes

INTRODUCTION

You work hard in your clinical nurse leader (CNL) position, improving patient outcomes by utilizing leadership skills, while collaborating with interdisciplinary teams. You identify gaps in care, determine best practice, guide teams in initiating projects that decrease falls, prevent infection and skin injury, improve communication practices, and much, much more. However, you have neglected to disseminate all of your wonderful achievements, so no one really knows the great things you have done in your practice. What you have been able to accomplish is relevant to the quality measures within your organization, and in many other areas of practice, and should be disseminated to others. Other nursing professionals and organizations can use your knowledge to create microsystems that are just as successful as yours. Dissemination is also a way of illustrating the value of the CNL in today's cost-constrained healthcare environments. This chapter discusses why dissemination is important and how to go about communicating your accomplishments.

After reading this chapter, you will be able to:

1. Identify the importance of dissemination
2. Examine opportunities for dissemination
3. Describe the elements of an abstract and how to give presentations

IMPORTANCE OF DISSEMINATION

There are many reasons to disseminate. Oermann and Hays (2018) state there are five main reasons to disseminate in publication, which includes "sharing ideas and expertise; disseminate evidence and findings of nursing research; for promotion, tenure, and personnel decisions; for development of one's own knowledge and skills; and for personal satisfaction" (p. 3). Nurses in some areas of practice, such as academia, are often required to publish their research and scholarly activities to attain tenure and maintain their positions. Nurses who work in the governmental policy arena may write to move agendas forward (Roush, 2017a). Clinical nurses, however, often concentrate their efforts on caring for patients and do not always think about presenting their work at conferences or writing for publication. Gobel (2018) states the reason nurses should publish their work is to "inform, educate, motivate and persuade" (p. 386). The work nurses do is of great importance to patient care and outcomes, and more nurses need to engage in dissemination. This is especially important for the CNL, not only to acknowledge what they do and what they can bring to healthcare but also in communicating this to others.

The CNL was developed in 2004 to address the gaps in care within the healthcare systems. However, there are still many organizations that either do not utilize them, utilize them in different positions, or have eliminated the position due to lack of positive measurable outcomes. The organizations that do utilize the CNL recognize the benefits and continue to embrace the role by expanding the CNL presence within their institutions. The CNLs from these organizations are those who are communicating what they bring to the table, and presenting to administrators, at conferences, and writing about their accomplishments.

Nursing as a whole has been lax in advocating for itself, which has been somewhat detrimental to the profession in the way of decision-making power, and recognition of what nursing brings to the overall healthcare system. Tyndall, Scott, and Caswell (2017) state that "clinical nurses are in pivotal positions to both share best practices, to influence healthcare reform and advance nursing science in hospital settings" (p. 522). The American Nurses Credentialing Center (ANCC) Magnet® Recognition Program® recognizes organizations that align strategic goals with nursing to improve patient outcomes (ANCC, n.d.). Organizations with Magnet status must demonstrate that they have supported nursing research and dissemination by clinical nurses, which illustrates the importance of dissemination by practicing point-of-care nurses (Tyndall et al., 2017).

Essential Facts

"The world is gradually recognizing that nursing really does matter. We also have to truly believe it ourselves" (Thorne, 2018, p. 3).

Presenting or publishing your work is not only beneficial to the profession but also a way to develop new skills and add to your resume. The knowledge that CNLs bring to healthcare is applicable in all types of settings, and career mobility throughout the healthcare system is easier when you have demonstrated undertakings beyond patient care. The CNL is known for their advanced patient care abilities, but if you are competing for a particular position, you need to set yourself apart from other applicants. Leading quality improvement initiatives and disseminating those results is great way of doing that.

HOW TO BEGIN

Many nurses feel they do not have anything to write about, or lack the time, ability, and resources to write for publication or present at conferences, when in reality, they just need assistance in developing ideas. Gobel (2018) suggests nurses should read journals in areas of interest to assist them in brainstorming ideas of their own activities that would be interesting to others. This author once noted an article on a particular learning strategy used by an educator teaching a CNL course. That same strategy was being used by this author but was never thought of in regard to writing about it in a journal. Often people get so caught up in performance of everyday work that the potential impact of what actually is being accomplished never comes to mind. When reading others' work, ask yourself if you are doing anything similar that may be of interest to others. What are you doing that is benefiting the patient and other nurses? What are the leading issues in healthcare and your patient population, and how are you addressing these challenges?

Finding a mentor to assist is often very helpful in coming up with ideas and writing. Discuss your work with managers, clinical nurse specialists, nurse practitioners, and other nurses within your organization to assist in developing ideas. If you established a rapport with past faculty members, set up an appointment to talk over your ideas with them. Often, it just takes looking at your work in a different perspective. Faculty often assist former students by sitting down and really questioning what they have been doing on their units. Again, what you may see as everyday work, others see as potential for dissemination. The project you performed in your educational program is often a great starting point. Many of this author's students have presented their projects at several different conferences because their topic is interesting in different areas of nursing.

It may also be helpful to begin with a group of nurses or even interdisciplinary teams in developing presentations and articles. In one organization, several CNLs worked together on a project focused on addressing the impact that long stay patients had within the medical units. These nurses had worked with an interdisciplinary team to develop patient-specific care plans to address the multiple needs of the patient. A faculty member assisted them in seeing that this was an extremely important initiative and should be disseminated. An abstract was developed (see abstract example in Exhibit 10.1), sent to the annual American Association of Colleges of Nursing (AACN) CNL Symposium, and was selected for a podium presentation. The presentation resulted in great discussion from the audience as other organizations have been dealing with the same issue. How these CNLs addressed the problem permitted others to gain insight as to how they might deal with their own organizational problems.

Essential Facts

While historically the 3Ps of dissemination included Posters, Presentations, and Papers, today's CNL can utilize a few more Ps, such as Podcasts, blogPosts, and social media Platforms.

Types of presentations and publishable works may include research, quality improvement projects, reviews of clinical articles, analysis of professional issues, opinions on healthcare topics, personal narratives on nursing, and patient experiences (Roush, 2017b).

Topics of interest vary, but fatigue, coping with stress, nurse resiliency, bullying, generational workplace differences, transitions to practice, and nurse turnover are often talked about problems or concerns. Shift work is also an important topic with recent concerns for patient well-being when nurses work 12 or more hours a day. Nurse wellness or lack of wellness is also a major talking point these days, as studies have shown that many nurses do not eat, sleep, or exercise as they should. Other topics may include interprofessional practice and how your unit or organization engages interprofessional communication and team work. Quality and safety initiatives such as reducing falls, hospital-acquired conditions, and rehospitalizations are also worth disseminating as most clinicians are working to improve in these areas. Roush (2017a) states that nursing is an art and science so what motivates you in your professional work can be written from your own personal vantage point through stories, which can be interesting and motivating to others.

WHERE TO DISSEMINATE

Administration

First and foremost, every CNL should maintain data and records related to their activities and outcomes within their particular microsystems. It is essential to communicate to administration your value to the organization. When developing budgets, organizations look at nursing positions as those that provide direct patient care and those that are supportive or administrative. Managers, assistant nurse managers, educators, and CNLs fall into the supportive or administrative group. When attempting to cut costs, the supportive roles are the ones that administration looks at to determine their worth and value to the organization.

With this in mind, the CNL must always be thinking about the importance of justifying worth by keeping records of achievements in patient care outcomes and nurse retention. This is especially important for areas such as falls, falls with injury, pressure injuries, hospital-acquired infection rates, and nurse turnover. What are your unit trends for these types of events? What initiatives have you put into place that has improved the outcomes in these areas? Also, be tracking length of stay and noting your efforts in managing transitions and discharge processes. Maintaining accurate records will allow you to communicate your worth and potentially retain your position.

Essential Facts

Be proactive! Schedule an annual professional presentation for your supervisor and other administrators to showcase your work. Present completed work, in-progress activities, and future plans, highlighting your financial and clinical impact on the organization.

Interorganizational Venues and Conferences

Some people are nervous about presenting in front of a group of people so it can be helpful to begin with a small audience such as in a staff meeting and then moving on to larger venues. Many larger organizations have monthly nursing presentations such as nursing grand rounds, where internal nurses present on a variety of relevant topics. Some organizations also have their own scholarship days where clinical nurses present posters on recent projects and initiatives. These are wonderful opportunities to disseminate your work among peers, which provide experience in presenting in a venue that may seem less stress inducing. If your organization does not have these types of opportunities, discuss the possibility of initiating them with administration as a means of enhancing professional development of clinical nurses.

There are many regional and national conferences focusing on different nursing specialties that host conferences. A listing of some of the organizations that host conferences can be found in Table 10.1. If you belong to a specialty organization, it is a good idea to provide your email address so you are kept up to date on events and conferences at which you could present. Pay attention to the dates of the conferences and the dates when abstract submissions are due. Abstract submissions are generally due several months in advance of the conference, and organizations will not accept abstracts after their posted date. If you have been working on a project that seems to coincide with an upcoming conference, create an abstract and title and send it to the conference committee. You will either be accepted or be declined. Not everyone is selected to every conference they submit. Either way, you are not out anything but your time and you have gained knowledge about how to write an abstract and will have it to start a new one for future submission.

Essential Facts

Nurses are lifelong learners, especially CNLs! They want to hear what you have to say.

Table 10.1

Organizational Conferences for Nurses and Nursing Specialties

American Association of Colleges of Nursing CNL Symposium Annual National Conference	https://www.aacnnursing.org
Clinical Nurse Leader Association Annual National CNLA conference	https://cnlassociation.org
American Academy of Hospice and Palliative Medicine Annual National Conference	http://aahpm.org/meetings/assembly
Society of Pediatric Nurses	www.pedsnurses.org
Association of Perioperative Registered Nurses Annual National Conference	https://www.aorn.org/join?utm _source=bing&utm_medium =search&utm_campaign =Membership_Prospecting _2019&utm_content=Explore
National Magnet Conference	https://www.nursingworld.org/ana
American Nurses Association Quality and Innovation Conference	http://anaqiconference.org
Oncology Nursing Society Congress	https://www.ons.org
National Association of Orthopaedic Nurses Annual Congress	www.orthonurse.org
Academy of Medical-Surgical Nurses Annual Conference	https://www.amsn.org
American Association of Critical-Care Nurses National Teaching Institute & Critical Care Exposition	https://www.aacn.org
American Holistic Nurses Association Annual Conference	https://www.ahna.org
Sigma Theta Tau	https://www.sigmanursing.org

TITLE AND ABSTRACT DEVELOPMENT

Developing a title and abstract is not difficult but can be time-consuming at times in attempting to choose the best words to convey the major aspects of your project or paper. The title is what people read first so it is a very important aspect in being accepted to a conference or having others read your article. A good title should express the message you want delivered in a summarizing manner relaying the "most interesting or novel aspects in order to attract the reader's attention" (Sturgeon & Ditadi, 2018, p. 1325). The title must also be long enough to convey your points but short enough to gain attention (Cook & Bordage, 2016). The readers you want to attract first are the abstract reviewers for the conference you wish to attend or reviewers for the journal in which you wish to publish. If you are sending the abstract to a conference committee, depending on the size of the conference, reviewers may have as many as 30 to 35 other abstracts to review, so it is important to write it in a way that peaks the reader's attention (Sturgeon & Ditadi, 2018). If you are working on an article abstract, it is often best to wait to write the title and abstract after you finish the article, as you can copy and paste different portions directly from the article text.

When forming the title, Tullu (2019) suggests writing three sentences describing your project, including the main information and subject. Once you have written the sentences, join them together and remove redundant words and information and then revise it further, making it "concise (about 10–15 words) and precise" (Tullu, 2019, p. S13). Precise refers to ensuring the title focuses on your project, study, or work. It is often a good idea to look at other journal articles and titles to see how different authors construct their titles. Cook and Bordage (2016) suggest avoiding "catchy, dramatic, fad or gimmicky titles ... because they are easily misinterpreted" (p. 1101). These authors also suggest making a list of key and related terms about the project and then create several titles using those terms. Ponder on the created titles, and ask others for their opinions to determine which one would fit best with your work.

Essential Facts

Do not let creating titles and abstracts block your writing! Many times, composing the final title of your work and writing the abstract occurs after you have completed your paper or presentation, allowing you to consider all of the information within your work.

Development of the abstract requires attention to the specific requirements of either the journal or the conference, as these may vary. If your abstract does not meet the requirements, it will not be published or read by the selection committee. When determining if your project aligns with the conference, identify the areas of interest. For example, the 2019 CNL Symposium sponsored by the AACN called for abstracts of projects that focused on the quadruple aim, CNL skill set in nontraditional settings, emerging trends in healthcare and education, improving outcomes in complex care environments with complex populations, and other such topics. A CNL wishing to present at this symposium would align with one of these categories and then write the abstract to highlight points of interest that are unique or novel to the subject while focusing on that area of interest for a greater chance of being accepted.

The length of your abstract is determined by the publication or conference. Abstracts are typically no more than 250 or 300 words. Most conferences and journals have electronic submission databases that will only permit a certain number of characters to be written, so you must stay within that number. The abstract is divided into four or five headings, which is also often dependent upon where you are submitting. Generally, abstracts should include the background issue, the problem that was addressed, the methods and/or interventions, a results section, and a conclusion. The conclusion may be written into the results section in some abstracts.

The background is addressing why you chose to address the problem or issue and why it is significant to either nursing, patient care and outcomes, or organizations. Highlight unique ways of addressing the issue. This would coincide with why you determined a change in practice was needed. For example, if you performed an evidence-based/quality improvement project on a problem with pressure injuries, you may explain how pressure injuries are a nursing quality indicator, which leads to increased pain and debilitation for the patient and longer lengths of stay for the organization and increased overall healthcare costs. The problem criterion addresses what the problem was in your particular microsystem that prompted further action or your initiative. You may have seen an increase in pressure injuries in the past several months that caused concern and warranted further action to be taken. There have been many initiatives to address pressure injuries, so if you are attempting to present on a common topic, make sure you highlight why your solution is different than others.

The methods section can also be listed as the "intervention" section and will describe how the project addressed the problem. In the example of pressure injuries, how the intervention addressed the increased pressure injuries would be discussed. A new turning regimen may have been initiated; therefore, you would discuss that initiative. The results section describes how the intervention improved the outcomes to the patient or the organization. If the project reduced pressure injuries by a certain percentage, that would be the results.

The American Association of Nursing has an annual Magnet conference, and its requirements are different than many other organizations. Instead of word counts, they require certain character counts, and the headings are also slightly different. Therefore, it is important to read and understand each organization's requirements to avoid extra work and possibly rejection.

The following abstracts provide examples of various methods of abstract and title development. Abstract Example 1 illustrates a CNL project improvement project within a large medical center written in a general abstract manner (Exhibit 10.1). Example 2 illustrates an EBP project abstract written for a Magnet conference (Exhibit 10.2), and Example 3 illustrates how a research study abstract could be written for a conference (Exhibit 10.3). These may help guide you in developing your own abstract. In the end, attempt to create a title and abstract that speaks to the goals of the conference or journal and include novel ideas of addressing the issue. Also, obtain insight from others who have written abstracts and have been accepted for either publication or conference presentations. Their insight will help you create a great title and abstract that will be accepted for poster or podium presentation or article submission.

Exhibit 10.1

Abstract Example 1: Following the General Abstract Formatting

Title:	CNL-Initiated Interdisciplinary Care Planning to Improve the Care of Long-Stay Patients in Acute Care Settings
Background:	Healthcare organizations are faced with increasing numbers of patients with complicated medical conditions. Discharge often requires interdisciplinary collaboration to ensure patients obtain services necessary to maintain optimal health. However, discharge for some patients lacking mental decision-making capacity, including some with behavioral issues, can be difficult. Individuals without family, friends, or legal representation may take months or even years to be discharged.
Problem:	A large academic medical center with four medical units has an average patient length of stay of 4 days for most patients. However, each unit has an average of five patients at any point in time considered long-stay patients, where their length of stay is anywhere from 35–400+ days. Healthcare professionals face many challenges caring for these patients in a safe, effective manner due to possible patient noncompliance, aggressive behaviors, and staff not understanding how to handle long-term patients.

Exhibit 10.1

Abstract Example 1: Following the General Abstract Formatting (*continued*)

Title:	CNL-Initiated Interdisciplinary Care Planning to Improve the Care of Long-Stay Patients in Acute Care Settings
Intervention:	Clinical nurse leaders (CNLs) and CNL students responded to these challenges by leading an initiative to develop interdisciplinary care plans in an attempt to meet the specific needs of individual long-stay patients. The care plans involve social services and ancillary professionals such as physical and occupational therapy, along with the medical teams and nursing. Team meetings facilitated by the CNLs develop and evaluate care plans that address common hospital risks such as pneumonia and falls, along with things such as opioid contracts for at risk patients, and limit setting efforts to decrease behavioral outbursts.
Results:	The establishment of specific interdisciplinary care plans has improved overall outcomes for the patients as well as improved staff morale by creating a safe, patient-specific experience and enabling staff to care for them in a safe effective manner. Since the initiation of these care plans, there has been a reduction in patient complications, outbursts, and elopement attempts.

Exhibit 10.2

Abstract Example 2: Magnet Conference

	Requirements
Topic: Evidence-based practice. Aligning unit-specific orientation with clinical experience	As patient acuities and nursing shortages increase, it becomes important to align education with clinical experience for each new nurse. Unit-specific education was developed and utilized, improving new nurse knowledge and preceptor satisfaction.
Purpose (what): Identify overall goal of the initiative [300]	Faced with a major influx of new nurses, and preceptors with varied skill level, standardized nurse education specific to a 36-bed inpatient unit was developed. The goal was to improve consistency of orientation education, perceive disease-specific knowledge, and increase preceptor satisfaction. **[298]**

(*continued*)

Exhibit 10.2

Abstract Example 2: Magnet Conference (*continued*)

	Requirements
Relevance/significance (why): Describe initiative's relevance and importance in context of the conference goal(s) and why the initiative was necessary [500]	As healthcare becomes more complex and specialized with increased patient acuity, it is important for new nurses to understand specific needs of particular patient populations. Studies have shown that new nurses lack overall confidence and skills for up to 1 year after graduation. Increasing their knowledge by providing additional educational support can improve critical thinking and patient outcomes and potentially decrease turnover rates through improved nurse satisfaction. [**482**]
Strategy and implementation (how): Describe the initiative actions and the process of implementation [1000]	An educational needs assessment was completed by clinical nurses, which identified knowledge gaps related to the pathophysiology and treatment of the unique patient population care for on the unit. Current evidence-based practice guidelines and literature were used to develop resources to address the identified needs and were provided to each nurse. They included information specific to the common disease processes and complications seen within the unit, including risk factors, signs/symptoms, diagnosis criteria, and treatment. Treatment information included common side effects for the nurse to know and confidently manage. A competency assessment and skills check-off sheet was developed and included to ensure each nurse received the same experiences and served as a guide for preceptors to determine additional learning needs. This helped to standardize the nurse's orientation to ensure each nurse is adequately prepared to safely care for the patients on the unit. [**974**]
Evaluation/outcomes (so what): Describe analytic findings and include actual evaluation data demonstrating the value of the	Surveys were completed preproject implementation and 8 weeks post by each new nurse using a Likert scale. Overall, there was dramatic improvement of 33%

Exhibit 10.2

Abstract Example 2: Magnet Conference (*continued*)

	Requirements
initiative change (success or failure) [400]	in the nurse's perceived understanding of each topic addressed, as well as an increase in preceptor satisfaction. The success of this evidence-based initiative has since led to replication in ambulatory clinics. [**365**]
Implications for practice (and now): Discuss specific implications for nursing practice. [300]	It is important to align education with clinical experiences to improve nurse competency and satisfaction. The development and utilization of specific education provides new nurses with a smooth transition to practice and ensures they can provide quality care to increasingly complex patients. [**292**]

Exhibit 10.3

Abstract Example 3: Research Study

Title:	We Won't Be Silos Anymore! Interprofessional Multipatient Clinical Simulation by Health Science Students, Designed to Change Practice.
Background:	Leading multidisciplinary teams including the client as part of the team is a recommended practice experience for clinical nurse leader (CNL) students (Wilcox, Rohrig, Nahikian-Nelms, & Robinson, 2018). Educational preparation for CNL students requires learning opportunities in team development that foster effective interprofessional communication and development of skills for advancing collaborative clinical reasoning skills. Acute care settings are dealing with turnover of staff nurses and other professionals, resulting in greater numbers of novice health professionals. The CNL must understand the knowledge base and critical thinking abilities of novices, as they manage teams, improve communication, and coordinate care to improve outcomes.
Method:	A descriptive study using mixed method design with pre- and postsimulation survey examined attitudes, confidence, and understanding of the other professionals' roles. Students engaged in a multidisciplinary simulation involving interprofessional rounds and collaborative care of two complex standardized patients. Over 400 health profession students from nursing, (including senior undergraduate, acute care

(continued)

Exhibit 10.3

Abstract Example 3: Research Study (*continued*)

Title:	**We Won't Be Silos Anymore! Interprofessional Multipatient Clinical Simulation by Health Science Students, Designed to Change Practice.**
	nurse practitioner, and CNL students), respiratory therapy, medical dietetics, physical therapy, occupational therapy, speech language pathology, medicine, and acute care nurse practitioner programs have completed a 2.5-hr simulation.
Objectives:	To create a climate of mutual respect and understanding, understand the roles and responsibilities of the other professions, develop interprofessional communication skills, and develop a multidisciplinary team plan of care to improve patient outcomes. CNL students were to identify the novice level of knowledge, clinical decision-making, and characteristics of critical thinking, as they manage care of patients.
Outcomes:	Participation in the simulations reflected a positive change in attitude and confidence. Postsurvey items indicated statistically significant ($p<.05$) improvement. CNL student responses were positive in learning novice characteristics as well as utilization of CNL roles to improve collaborative clinical reasoning. An added benefit that CNL students noted was the ability to educate student professionals on roles and responsibilities of the CNL.

PRESENTATIONS AND PUBLICATIONS

Poster Presentations

Following acceptance to present at a conference, you will need to put forth effort in creating your presentation, whether it is a poster or podium format. Christenbery and Latham (2013) state that a great poster may take up to 8 weeks to create, so begin early in planning. You will also need to consider the time that is required for printing. Check with your organization or college, as they may have poster templates with their logo and printing services available, which will decrease potential costs. Poster templates are generally PowerPoint slides that are formatted with poster sections. The top will have a title section where you will include the title along with your name and any organizational affiliation. Below the title are three or four columns to enter text and graphics.

Be sure to check with the organization through which you have been accepted to present, as requirements vary. Some conferences require portrait format rather than the traditional landscape format, and specific measurements may be required. Posters can be either laminated paper or cloth. Cloth posters may be slightly more expensive, but if flying to a conference, it is much easier to fold and place in your suitcase rather than navigating airports and planes with your poster.

Besides the physical size and layout of the poster, conferences may have different requirements for headings within the poster. Some conferences require that you use headings that are typically used for research such as introduction/background, problem, methods, results, and implications for nursing or discussion, whereas others may require more general headings such as problem, clinical initiative, outcomes and recommendations, and conclusion (Christenbery & Latham, 2013). Depending upon your topic and your project, you could include headings such as interventions, procedures, themes, and limitations if they fit within the poster size. The poster is a summation of your project; do not attempt to write everything within the poster as you are highlighting the important aspects of your work.

Essential Facts

During poster presentations, the poster draws others in to view your work; you keep them there by presenting additional information of interest. The goal is to leave positive impressions and interesting ideas with viewers. And, of course, your contact information!

When creating the poster, begin with the headings and use bullet points to highlight points instead of writing in paragraph form. You do not want to overwhelm the reader with words. The AACN (n.d.-b) states that the poster should be readable at a distance of 5 feet and the actual text of the poster should be approximately one quarter of the poster space. Graphs and charts are a wonderful addition to all posters and can really display data much better than words. Graphics and photographs also add and permit a visualization of how you performed the initiative. You want to highlight the important facts but you do not want to overwhelm the reader. Pedwell, Hardy, and Rowland (2016) state that excess information should be avoided to create a sense of coherence within the poster and anything that distracts the reader is considered "noise." Excess words or too many graphics could be considered noise and therefore distracting to the reader.

Your poster should have balance and be aesthetically pleasing to the reader. Select colors, fonts, and visuals that are pleasing to the eye and understandable from a distance. Pedwell, Hardy, and Rowland (2016) created fictional posters for their students to assist them in learning how to create effective posters. These examples provide a little levity to the topic and prevent hard feelings from others who produced a poster that was lacking. You will find these posters in Exhibits 10.4, 10.5, and 10.6. These nicely illustrate the differences in appearance with wording, illustrations, and graphs.

Conferences often have poster-viewing sessions where the presenter can discuss their work with viewers. You may want to create a handout to provide viewers who stop at your poster during the viewing or for additional information when you are not there. The handout may consist of a smaller version of your poster or an outline of points with references. Be sure to also prepare a short summary of your poster to discuss with viewers. There are often questions asked about how the project was performed, what obstacles existed, and if the work is sustainable. You may also want to provide viewers with your business card in case they would like to contact you for further information at a later date.

Besides presenting at the conference, poster sessions are a great way of networking, learning new information, and seeing what others are doing in the way of patient care. Be proud of your work and accomplishment in being accepted to the conference. You have done a great job, and now is your time to let everyone know.

Podium Presentations

Podium presentations will most likely take more time and effort in the preparation phase than a poster. You will actually be presenting the information to an audience, and the slide design, as well as how you present the information, will affect the manner in which you are received. When creating a podium presentation, there are some key points to consider. First you will need to consider the audience. You have been accepted because your information aligns with the topics and purpose of the conference. Make sure you focus on the goals when developing your presentation. For example, an objective of the conference may be on interdisciplinary practice. Your abstract mentioned that you worked with interdisciplinary teams, which is most likely one of the reasons you were accepted to present. In your mind, however, your work may be important because of the outcomes you achieved for your particular population of patients. To align your presentation with the audience and the goals of the conference, you should focus on how you incorporated interdisciplinary team members into achieving your outcomes.

Exhibit 10.4

Excellent Poster

Pug farts are a viable control method for *Mortuus ovis*

Rhianna Pedwell[a], James Hardy[a], Susan Rowland[a]
[a]The University of Queensland, St Lucia QLD 4072, Australia

1. THE NEED FOR ZOMBIE CONTROL

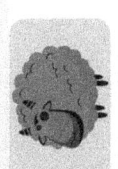

Zombie sheep hordes have threatened human safety for half a decade, with an estimated 67% of all domesticated sheep infected globally as of 2014 [1]. As yet, no viable control methods exist for the outbreaks, with many resorting to the use of automatic or hand-held weaponry [2]. A recent study by Dettman, I (2013), showed that Pug (*Canis lupus familiaris*) farts (when labeled 'inebo' are +*ve* effective in killing *Mortuus ovis* infections). Post mortems recorded the hydrogen sulphide in pug farts had acted as a neurotoxin on the zombie herds, effectively a 'shot to the head' in small form [3].

This study represents the first attempt to optimise the pug fart dose for use on current and future *M. ovis* outbreaks. Preliminary data showed feeds high in sulphur to be ideal for producing pug farts high in hydrogen sulphide — a key ingredient for keeping our zombie terrorism across a sample population (n = 4). We predicted feeding pugs a high-egg diet would cause them to produce farts capable of causing *M. ovis* neutral cell damage.

2. FART COLLECTION & ANALYSIS

n = 12 Pugs fed NED, LED, or HED for 3 days
↓
Farts collected in Olsor-Vac & condensed
↓
Condensed fart sample applied to Staffometer   Fart extract applied to *M. ovis* neural cell culture

Table 1: Daily Diet Fed to Test Animals

Treatment Group	Eggs Fed	Daily Diet Standard Diet
No-egg Diet (NED), n = 4	0	Water supply, 250g dry food
Low-egg Diet (LED), n = 4	1	Water supply, 250g dry food
High-egg Diet (HED), n = 4	3	Water supply, 250g dry food

3. OUTCOMES OF FART ANALYSIS

- Pugs fed high-egg diet produced most farts with 25.8 ml
- Low and no-egg diet Pugs produced 8.8±2.95 ml farts
- Pugs fed high-egg diet produced 'super' smelly [4] farts with 18.7 intensity units (IU) of sulphur smell [5]
- Low-egg and no-egg diet Pug farts negative (12.8±3) and 'really' (6.5 IU) smelly
- High-egg diet farts lethal to *M. ovis* neural cells *in vitro*
- Low-egg and no-egg diets not lethal to *M. ovis* neural cells

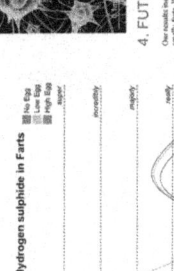

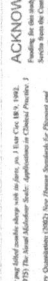

Figure 3. *M. ovis* Neural Cell Imaging Results. *M. ovis* neural cell cultures before treatment with 10 μl of fart extract from; A) NED pug fart extract (Image A), and after 1 hour incubation in Image B). Neuroregenerative could not be seen in HEF cell culture line.

4. FUTURE USE OF FARTS

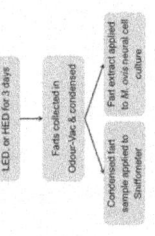

Our results indicate pugs fed on a high-egg diet produce a large volume of lethally smelly farts. We have shown that hydrogen sulphide at a small volume of at least 18.7 (super smelly) is a viable option for inducing lethal neural cell death in *M. ovis*. The production costs associated with harvesting farts from Pugs, however, make this method far from economically sustainable. Further limitations of the study include long processing times, and potential for inconsistent results. We suggest an extension of this research would investigate farts that could lead to the development of Pug farts as a viable lethal factor *in vivo*. In the future, we hope to test this method on *in vivo* models, and bring humanity one step closer to ending the zombie plague.

ACKNOWLEDGEMENTS

Funding for this study was provided by GDLC grant KT2003472. We would like to acknowledge Ass. Santica Yum, Chnelyn B. van Stassen, and Arizona Fonamura, who provided cell lines. We are grateful to Wolfgang Baird Gregin for his assistance with use of animal subjects.
Rebecca Lee assists A, Mam Lee (contents B, CC BY-SA).

REFERENCES

1. Perseus, I (2019) *M. pug lethal zombie sheep with incisors, etc.* J Xoat Ctrl 18(1): 1982.
2. Pedlingtone, S, Y, I (1975) *The Small Melodious Smile: Applications to Clinical Practise.* J Med Mani 4, 5, 476.
3. Department of Sensory Quantitation (2002) *New Human Standards for Fibroscent and zombie sewerage* J Med Mam Seep, 7, 11, 210-255.
4. Pedlingtone, S, Y, I (1975) *The Small Melodious Smile: Applications to Clinical Practise.* J Med Mani 4, 5, 476.
5. Dettman, I (2014) *Five Roses fly after the Outbreak: How are we dealing with the zombie outbreak?* (Objection: Odnoet, Request published online).

Source: Reproduced from Pedwell, R., Hardy, J., & Rowland, S. (2016) Effective visual design and communication practices for research posters: Exemplars based on the theory and practice of multimedia learning and rhetoric. *Biochemistry and Molecular Biology Education, 45*(3), 249–261. doi:10.1002/bmb.21034

Exhibit 10.5

Average Poster

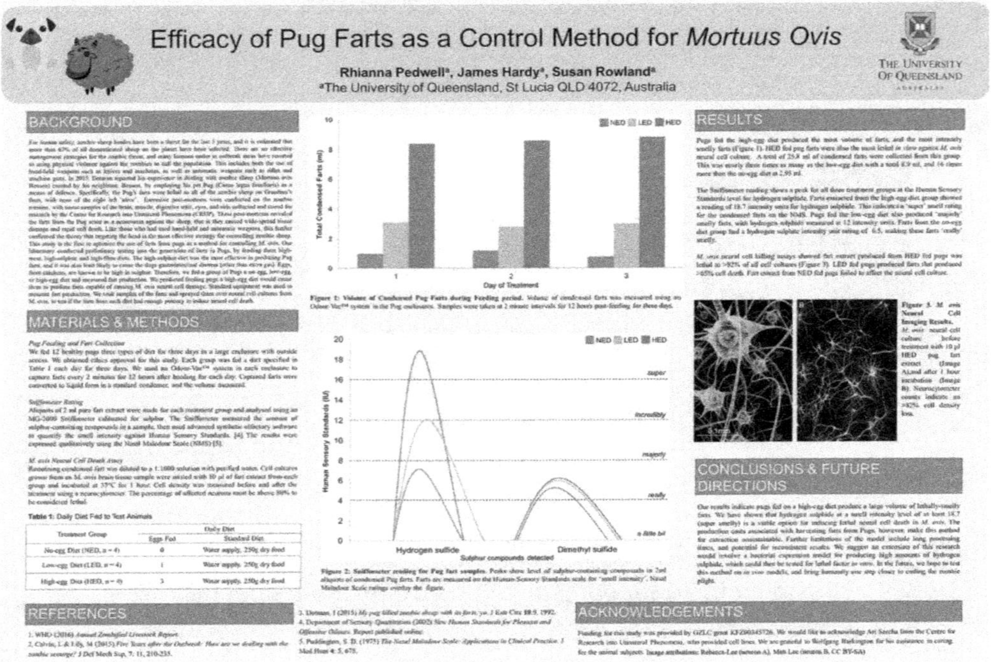

Source: Reproduced from Pedwell, R, Hardy, J., & Rowland, S. (2016) Effective visual design and communication practices for research posters: Exemplars based on the theory and practice of multimedia learning and rhetoric. *Biochemistry and Molecular Biology Education, 45*(3), 249–261. doi:10.1002/bmb.21034

Exhibit 10.6

Terrible Poster

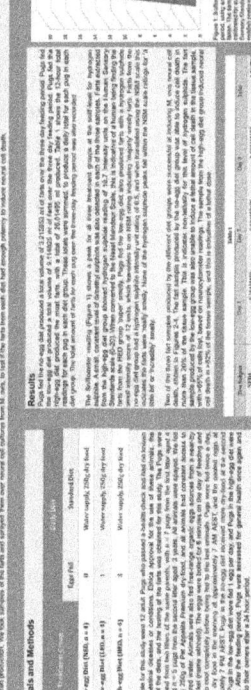

Source: Reproduced from Pedwell, R., Hardy, J., & Rowland, S. (2016) Effective visual design and communication practices for research posters: Exemplars based on the theory and practice of multimedia learning and rhetoric. *Biochemistry and Molecular Biology Education*, 45(3), 249–261. doi:10.1002/bmb.21034. https://iubmb.onlinelibrary.wiley.com/doi/epdf/10.1002/bmb.21034; https://iubmb.onlinelibrary.wiley.com/doi/full/10.1002/bmb.21034.

Be sure to note the allotted time you will have to present. The length of the presentation may vary with the conference, but typically, presenters present for anywhere from 20 minutes to one or one and a half hours. Generally, you should figure one slide per minute when creating your slides. You do not want to rush through your presentation, so attempt to keep the slides to a minimum. Also keep in mind that the slides are there for engagement purposes and are not meant to be read word for word.

The design of your slides will play a major role in engaging others when presenting. The text should be in bullet form and not written as a paragraph. If you have too many words, the audience will read the slide instead of listening to what you have to say. The font should be large enough to be seen in the back of the room and should be a standard text without italics to make it easier to read. Reekers (2010) states that sans serif font should be used for titles, serif font should be used for bullets and body of the text, and sans serif font is best for charts and tables. It is best to limit the amount of information on each slide; the general rule is no more than eight lines per slide (AACN, 2018). As with a poster, charts, graphs, photos, and even humor will add to your discussion. Allow time for questions at the end of the presentation; this may vary from 5 to 10 minutes.

Essential Facts

Engaging you audience is key during podium presentations, making the first few seconds of your talk the most critical. Consider using a pointed question, shocking statistic, unusual visual, upbeat music, or any other attention-getting idea to start!

There are several different methods in how you organize the information. Reeker (2010) suggests using a chronological, problem, case study, or knowledge format. A chronological format takes you through steps. You would discuss how one step follows another, which would be an excellent way to discuss a project from start to finish. The problem format begins with the identified problem and impact of the problem. You state the problem, its impact, what you did to determine solutions, and then outcomes from those solutions. Case studies are great ways of engaging the audience and can add to your presentation. You can discuss your initiatives utilizing the patient problems that led you to initiate your project. Often, the audience will have had similar patient experiences and want to discuss your methods further following the presentation. The knowledge format is summarizing an innovative idea or information. It may be on a new product, technique, or procedure that you found useful in improving patient care or patient care outcomes. Reeker (2010) suggests that this format should be developed in a way that allows the audience to easily follow, digest, and remember the information.

Be sure to rehearse your talk several times. It is often good to present to another person to obtain feedback regarding any small habits that might distract the audience such as saying "um" often or moving too much or too little or anything else that may interfere with getting your message across. You want to know your content and do your best but do not worry about making a mistake during your presentation. Most often, everyone has a moment during a talk that gets them off track just move on or make light of it. Having some humor in your presentation will just lighten the mood a little.

Publications

Writing for publication is the best method of disseminating your work to a large audience. Conferences are very good, but the audience is limited to those attending. Articles reach a larger population and permit people from different healthcare backgrounds to learn from your work. If you have presented a project at a conference, either podium or poster presentation, this will provide you with the basis of the article. You have organized your thoughts within your presentation, so now all you have to do is write it in a manuscript format.

The writing process can seem difficult and time-consuming, but preparation can ease the process. Too often, nurses begin writing projects and never finish them because they have not made it a priority. It may help to write with a group of colleagues, but if that is not possible, attempt to find a mentor to assist you in writing and keep you on track. Nurse leaders within your organization who have published can be very helpful in getting you started. Set a due date for yourself for when you want different parts of the paper to be completed and stick to that timeline. Roush (2017a) suggests reading different articles to become familiar with the structure of journal articles, write regularly by setting time aside just for writing, and set up a space and time to write. Another suggestion is to read articles from different journals to provide insight to the type of information being written about, the style and structure of different journals, and the length of typical articles published in different journals (Wood, 2018). Once you have determined the journal to pursue, review their guidelines as each journal varies in their requirements on subjects, formatting, and length of articles. Following these suggestions will assist you in getting started and completing your writing project. A list of common journals and their websites is listed in Table 10.2. The last entry in the table provides a larger listing of journals that you may find useful in your search.

When developing your article, you should consider a general format that includes the abstract, an introduction, the main body of the paper, and conclusion (Wood, 2018). If your paper discusses a research or a quality improvement project, you should include sections within your body on the methods and results. The results section would include any statistical analysis you may have done. The conclusion would include a discussion on your finding and implications for further research or relevant practice changes that may strengthen the initiative.

Table 10.2

Common Nursing Journals and Websites

Journal	Website
Nursing Outlook	https://www.nursingoutlook.org
Journal of Cardiovascular Nursing	https://journals.lww.com/jcnjournal/pages/default.aspx
Journal of Nursing Care Quality (Official Journal of the Clinical Nurse Leader Association)	https://journals.lww.com/jncqjournal/pages/default.aspx
Nurse Education Today	https://www.journals.elsevier.com/nurse-education-today
Journal of Professional Nursing	https://www.journals.elsevier.com/journal-of-professional-nursing
American Journal of Nursing	https://journals.lww.com/ajnonline/pages/default.aspx
Oncology Nursing Journals	https://www.ons.org/journals
Holistic Nursing Practice	https://journals.lww.com/hnpjournal/pages/default.aspx
The Journal of Continuing Education in Nursing	https://www.healio.com/nursing/journals/jcen/submit-an-article
Journal of Nursing Administration	https://journals.lww.com/jonajournal/pages/default.aspx
NursingCenter	https://www.nursingcenter.com/articles-publications/all-journals

For quality improvement projects, there are guidelines that will help you in implementing your project as well as writing an article surrounding your work. These guidelines are called SQUIRE 2.0 Guidelines, which stands for Standards for Quality Improvement Reporting Excellence and can be found at www.squire-statement.org/index.cfm?fuseaction=page.viewpage&pageid=471. This is a very useful site as it walks you through the thought process of what you did and how you did it so you can write it in a complete manner. If you are writing about research that you performed, you may want to view the recommendations from the International Committee of Medical Journal Editors (ICMJE) at www.icmje.org. This committee provides a downloadable article discussing the recommendations for the reporting and publication of scholarly work within medical journals and is similar to the SQUIRE Guidelines in that it discusses important information regarding how to write the article (ICMJE, 2018).

When writing your paper, ensure that you are writing it using proper writing style and grammar. Avoid writing in first person, and use correct word tense and verb agreement, and other grammatical considerations. Make sure you know which format the journal requires, such as APA (American Psychological Association) or AMA (American Medical Association), as these styles differ, and it may be difficult to rewrite your article later in the correct format. Cite all of your references correctly, and limit the number of direct quotes you use; it is always best to paraphrase as much as possible. Proofread your paper several times, and have others read it to provide you with their insight. Attempt to have someone who has already published read your paper and even assist you through the writing process. Many advanced practice nurses, administrators, and faculty have published and are often willing to assist others in the publishing process.

There are many articles and books on the writing process that may assist you in getting started and move forward with your writing. A text that many find helpful is Oermann and Hays (2018). Dr. Oermann and Hays are authors very familiar with the writing process; Dr. Oermann is also a journal editor and has been assisting others in publishing for a number of years. The *American Journal of Nursing* has published a collection of writing resource articles that highlight how to navigate the many phases of the writing process. These articles can be found at https://journals.lww.com/ajnonline/pages/collectiondetails.aspx?TopicalCollectionId=39.

If you have access to a library database, you can search for other articles that may be helpful, as there have been many published.

Clinical Nurse Leader Vignette 10.1: Increasing Dissemination Confidence

Melissa was a student in her final CNL practicum. Her project focused on compassion fatigue and resiliency of nurses within an intensive care setting. She was very passionate about the problem as she found that compassion fatigue affected many nurses in acute care settings, especially intensive care settings. The problem of compassion fatigue ultimately affects the care provided to patients. Her main goal of the project was to develop interventions that would increase resiliency and thereby reduce compassion fatigue, while educating the nurses to the problem and methods to address it.

Melissa, however, had little experience in presenting information and did not have confidence in her presentation skills. Her preceptor and instructor mentored her on how to develop a presentation and deliver an effective speech. She practiced her talk in front of her preceptor and instructor and was provided feedback on what she did well and how she might improve. She took the feedback and worked hard to improve her presentation style.

Melissa gained enough confidence through her efforts to present her project to a small group of staff during a staff meeting in her precepted site. She received excellent feedback from the group, which increased her confidence. She then took the presentation to her place of employment, and again received excellent feedback, and identified nurses who were actually using her intervention throughout their shifts. Melissa not only gained confidence in presenting, but she was able to see the difference she was making through her teaching, which impacted the nurses. She not only gained confidence in her presentation style, but with each presentation, she received further acknowledgment that her project was important and helpful to nurses and in the long run improved patient care.

Following graduation, Melissa developed an abstract, with faculty assistance to a local nursing conference and was accepted for a poster presentation. She then went on to submit abstracts on her own to two major national conferences. She was accepted at both with one being a podium presentation. With each presentation, Melissa was able to gain further confidence while providing essential skills to others to prevent a major issue within nursing: compassion fatigue. Melissa is now working on an article with a major nursing journal.

References

American Association of Colleges of Nursing. (2018). *Slide design tips*. Retrieved from https://www.aacnnursing.org/Portals/42/Professional-Development/Conferences/AACN-Slide-Design-Tips.pdf

American Association of Colleges of Nursing. (n.d.). *Recommendations for effective abstract poster presentations*. Retrieved from https://www.aacnnursing.org/Portals/42/Professional-Development/Conferences/Poster-Recommendations.pdf

American Nurses Credentialing Center. (n.d.). *ANCC Magnet Recognition Program*®. Retrieved from https://www.nursingworld.org/organizational-programs/magnet/

Christenbery, T. L., & Latham, T. G. (2013). Creating effective scholarly posters: A guide for DNP students. *Journal of the American Association of Nurse Practitioners, 25*, 16–23. doi:10.1111/j.1745-7599.2012.00790.x

Cook, D. A., & Bordage, G. (2016). Twelve tips on writing abstracts and titles: How to get people to use and cite your work. *Medical Teacher, 38*(11), 1100–1104. doi:10.1080/0142159X.2016.1181732

Gobel, B. H. (2018). A clinical practice perspective on publishing in oncology nursing. *Seminars in Oncology Nursing, 34*(4), 386–392. doi:10.1016/j.soncn.2018.09.007

International Committee of Medical Journal Editors. (2018). *Recommendations for the conduct, reporting, editing, and publication of scholarly work in medical journals*. Retrieved from http://www.icmje.org/icmje-recommendations.pdf

Oermann, M. H., & Hays, J. C. (2018). *Writing for publication in nursing* (4th ed.). New York, NY: Springer Publishing Company.

Pedwell, R. K., Hardy, J. A., & Rowland, S. L. (2016). Effective visual design and communication practices for research posters: Exemplars based on the theory and practice of multimedia learning and rhetoric. *Biochemistry and Molecular Biology Education, 45*(3), 249–261. doi:10.1002/bmb.21034

Reekers, J. A. (2010). *Presenting at medical meetings*. New York, NY: Springer-Verlag.

Roush, K. (2017a). Becoming a published writer. How to create a writing life and tips on getting started. *American Journal of Nursing, 117*(3), 63–66. doi:10.1097/01.NAJ.0000520256.42212.fc

Roush, K. (2017b). What types of articles to write. A review of different journal articles and what editors are looking for. *American Journal of Nursing, 117*(5), 68–71. doi:10.1097/01.NAJ.0000516278.97098.02

Sturgeon, C. M., & Ditadi, A. (2018). Let me speak! A reviewers' guide to writing a successful meeting abstract. *Stem Cell Reports, 11*(6), 1324–1326. doi:10.1016/J.STEMCR.2018.11.016

Thorne, Sally. (2018). In search of our collective voice. *Nursing Inquiry, 25*, e12266. doi:10.1111/nin.12266

Tullu, M. S. (2019). Writing the title and abstract for a research paper: Being concise, precise, and meticulous is the key. *Saudi Journal of Anesthesia, 13*, S12–S17. doi:10.4103/sja.SJA_685_18

Tyndall, D. E., Scott, E. S., & Caswell, N. I. (2017). Factors facilitating publication by clinical nurses in a magnet hospital. *The Journal of Nursing Administration, 47*(10), 522–526. doi:10.1097/NNA.0000000000000525

Wilcox, J., Rohrig, L., Nahikian-Nelms, M., & Robinson, M. (2018, February). *We won't be silos anymore! Inter-professional multi-patient clinical simulation by health science students, designed to change practice.* Poster session presented at the CNL Summit & Master's Education Conference, Garden Grove, CA.

Wood, C. (2018). Writing for publication: Sharing your clinical knowledge and skills. *British Journal of Community Nursing, 23*(1), 20–23. doi:10.12968/bjcn.2018.23.1.20

Index

AACN. *See* American Association of Colleges of Nursing
AAFP. *See* American Academy of Family Physicians
abstract, 176, 178
   background, 181
   development, 179–182
   examples, 182–186
   length, 181
   Magnet conference, 183–185
   methods/interventions section, 181
   problem criterion, 181
   research study, 185–186
   results section, 181
action plan, 86
active listening, 19, 53, 129, 164
acute care, 3, 36
   documentation, 128–129
   patients, 62
   processes, 68
   professionals, 63, 66
   purpose of, 58
   readmissions, 126
   role of CNLs in, 21–22
administration, 11, 27
   and dissemination, 177–178
   staff, 54
advocacy, 157–158
   CNL networking structure, 167
   collaborative, 167
   patient, 158–162
   plan, 167
   professional nursing, 162–171
   spontaneous, 163
Agency for Healthcare Research and Quality, 122
alendronate sodium, 134
AMA. *See* American Medical Association
ambulatory care
   patients, 61–62
   processes, 68
   professionals, 63
   purpose of, 57–58
   role of CNLs in, 22
American Academy of Family Physicians (AAFP), 23, 57
American Association of Colleges of Nursing (AACN), 1, 3, 15, 21, 79, 135, 158, 159
   clinical nurse leader roles, 8
   CNL implementation task force, 163
   CNL Symposium, 176, 180–181
   poster presentation requirements, 187
American Association of Nursing, 182
American Journal of Nursing, 194
American Medical Association (AMA), 194

American Nurses Association (ANA), 122, 123
American Nurses Credentialing Center (ANCC), 175
American Psychological Association (APA), 194
American Society of Healthcare Engineering (ASHE), 61
amiodarone, 134
ANA. *See* American Nurses Association
ANCC. *See* American Nurses Credentialing Center
APA. *See* American Psychological Association
ASHE. *See* American Society of Healthcare Engineering
authoritarian leadership, 43

budget for change project, 151
Bundled Payments for Care Improvement Advanced, 122
butterfly effect, 38

Care Transitions Intervention (CITI), 124
CAS. *See* complex adaptive systems
case-controlled studies, 84
case studies, 191
cause and effect diagrams, 115
CCM. *See* Chronic Care Model
Centers for Disease Control and Prevention, 113
Centers for Medicare and Medicaid Services (CMS), 104, 122
cerebral vascular accident (CVA), 128
certified nurse practitioners, 12
change, 47, 139–140
  barriers, identification of, 148
  commitment to, 150
  communication of need for, 148–150
  EBP, implementation of, 86
  leadership, readying for, 142–143
  need in healthcare, 140–141
  process, implementation of, 150–151
  project
    implementation timeline, 151
    tools for, 151
  shifting healthcare paradigms, 144
  sustaining, 152–153
  theory, choosing, 143–147
chaos theory, 37–38, 52
charter, 150–151
Chronic Care Model (CCM), 125
chronological format, 191
CINAHL, 83
CIs. *See* confidence intervals
CITI. *See* Care Transitions Intervention
client advocate, CNL as, 7, 23
Clinical Nurse Leader Association, 15
clinical nurse leaders (CNLs), 1, 174
  benefits to organizations, 2
  coordination of care, 123
  creation of need for, 10–11
  definition of, 1–2
  employment of, 3–4
  financial impacts of, 55
  and professional nursing roles, differences between, 11–12
  rationale for, 2–3
  resources, 14
  role(s), 7–9, 163
    AACN, 8
    initiation of, 4–5
    management of, 24–27
clinical nurse specialists, 12
clinician, CNL as, 7, 161
cloth posters, 187
CMS. *See* Centers for Medicare and Medicaid Services
CNLs. *See* clinical nurse leaders
Cochrane Database of Systematic Reviews, 83
cohort studies, 84
collaboration, 4, 20, 25, 129, 135, 161
  in emergency care, 22
  with organizations, 167
communication, 18, 54
  and coordination of care, 127–129

interprofessional, 149
and medication mismanagement, 133
of need for change, 148–150
nonverbal, 130
plan, 149–150, 151
community
community health settings, role of CNLs in, 23–24
involvement, 166
microsystems, 160, 166
professional nursing advocacy within, 165–167
resources, 22, 125, 127
complex adaptive systems (CAS), 37–41, 159
leader characteristics in, 46
vs. traditional systems, 41
complex environments, leadership within, 45–47
complexity science, 37
conferences, 178–179
podium presentations, 189–191
poster presentations, 186–189, 190
confidence intervals (CIs), 85
conversational questions, 130
coordination of care, 121, 122, 159
challenges and strategies for, 127–135
communication, 127–129
definition of, 123
health literacy, 131
interdisciplinary team management, 135
on medical unit, 135–136
medication management, 133–135
patient-centered care, 129–131
readmissions, analyzing, 126–127
social determinants of health, 132
transition of care models, 124–125
critical appraisal for evidence, 84–85
culture
mircosystem, 54–55, 56
embedding change into, 152–153
organizational, 169
CUS (concerned, uncomfortable, safety) tool, 127
CVA. *See* cerebral vascular accident

Dartmouth Institute Microsystem Academy, 22
data, 111–112
collection/analysis, QI projects, 113–115
sources and types of, 111–113
databases
for healthcare research, 83
quality improvement, 113
Deming, William Edwards, 106–107
Deming cycle. *See* Plan, Do, Study, Act (PDSA) cycle
democratic leadership, 43
DIEP acronym, 143
diffusion of innovation theory, 145–146
discharge of patients
and communication, 128
delay in, 39–40
and medications, 133, 134–135
summaries, 128
disconfirmation, 140–141
dissemination, 173
administration, 177–178
beginning, 175–177
confidence, increasing, 194–195
importance of, 174–175
international venues/ conferences, 178–179
podium presentations, 189–191
poster presentations, 186–189, 190
publications, 192–194
title and abstract development, 179–186
topics of interest, 177
types of presentations and publishable works, 176
DMAIC (define, measure, analyze, improve, control), 107–108

Donabedian, Avedis, 105, 106
Donabedian model of quality assurance, 105–106
dosages of medications, 133

EBP. *See* evidence-based practice
EBSCO, 83
ECFs. *See* extended care facilities
educator, CNL as, 7
electronic medical records (EMRs), 112, 114, 128–129
elevator speech, 13, 20
emergency care, 39–40
　processes, 68
　professionals, 63
　purpose of, 57–58
　role of CNLs in, 22
EMRs. *See* electronic medical records
environment
　complex environments, leadership within, 45–47
　healthy work environments, 18, 163
　and patient outcomes, 80
　and wellness, 162
Environmental Protection Agency (EPA), 26
EPA. *See* Environmental Protection Agency
evidence-based practice (EBP), 24
　barriers, management of, 90–92
　change, implementation of, 86
　committees, 91–92
　critical appraisal for evidence, 84–85
　definition of, 81
　evaluation of outcomes and dissemination, 86
　historical perspective of, 80–81
　initiatives, in acute cardiac unit, 92–93
　models and resources, 87–90
　and patient preferences, 81
　PICOT question, 82–83
　process measures, 86
　project, abstract, 183–185
　relevance of evidence to practice, 81–82
　searching for evidence, 83–84
evidence-informed decision-making (McMaster University), 89–90
experienced nurses, transition into CNL role, 20
extended care facilities (ECFs), 125, 127, 128

failure mode and effects analysis (FMEA), 110–111
fishbone diagrams. *See* cause and effect diagrams
5P assessment, 26, 28–29, 56, 71–75
　patients, 58–62
　patterns, 69–70
　processes, 66–68
　professionals, 62–66
　purpose, 56–58
5 Why process, 110
flowcharts, 108, 116
FMEA. *See* failure mode and effects analysis
follow-up care, 131, 132, 134–135
formulary medications, 134
fragmentation of care, 158–160
frontline staff, 53, 61, 69, 150

Gantt charts, 116–117
global level advocacy, 169–171
goals
　metric-based, 54
　microsystem needs, 27
　organizational, 27
　prioritization, 30–31
　professional needs, 25
Guided Care Model, 124

handoff communication, 127
HCUP. *See* healthcare cost and utilization project
health literacy, 131
health nursing, 161

healthcare cost and utilization project (HCUP), 113
healthcare organizations
 current practices within, 104
 and quality improvement, 105
healthcare-related infections, 54
healthcare settings, CNL role within, 21
 acute care, 21–22
 community health settings, 23–24
 emergency/ambulatory care, 21–22
 primary care, 23
healthcare system(s)
 complexity of, 37–41
 connection to outside entities, 40
 evolution of, 36–37
 interactions and relationships in, 39–40
 navigation of, 160–161
 nonlinearity of, 38–39
 systems thinking, 40
 unpredictability of, 38
healthy work environments (HWEs), 18, 163
high-reliability organizations (HROs), 104
home care, 24
Home Health Model of Care Transitions, 125
horizontal leadership, 46–47
HROs. *See* high-reliability organizations
HWEs. *See* healthy work environments

ICMJE. *See* International Committee of Medical Journal Editors
IHI. *See* Institute for Healthcare Improvement
information manager, CNL as, 7, 9, 54, 160
Institute for Healthcare Improvement (IHI), 117, 118, 133
Institute of Medicine (IOM), 2, 129

aims for healthcare quality, 104
Crossing the Quality Chasm report, 80
INTERACT Model, 125
interdisciplinary communication, 127
interdisciplinary teams
 and dissemination, 176
 management, 135
International Committee of Medical Journal Editors (ICMJE), 193
international venues/conferences, 178
interprofessional communication, 149
interrater reliability, 114
IOM. *See* Institute of Medicine
Iowa Model, 87–89

Joanna Briggs Institute, 83
John Hopkins Evidence-Based Practice Model, 87, 97–101
Johns Hopkins Center for Evidence-Based Practice, 87
Johns Hopkins University, 124
journal clubs, 91
journal writing, 17, 24
journals, 175, 192, 193

knowledge format, 191
knowledge workers, 41–42, 45

laissez-faire leadership, 43–44
leadership, 36
 change leadership, readying for, 142–143
 characteristics, 46
 within complex environments, 45–47
 hematologic oncology unit, 47–48
 horizontal, 46–47
 reflection plan, 142–143
 relationship with employees, 42
 styles, 42–44
 traditional, 42–45

Lean Six Sigma, 107–108
learning anxiety, 141
level of evidence, 83
Lewin, Kurt, 145, 147, 150, 152
lifelong learner, CNL as, 9
linear systems, 38
Lippett, Ronald, 146, 147, 150
literature search, 83–84
long-term care
    patients, 62
    processes, 68
    professionals, 66
    purpose of, 58
long-term goals
    microsystem needs, 27
    professional needs, 25

Magnet-designated hospitals, 91
Magnet® Recognition Program®, 175
managers, 11
    microsystem, 53–54
marketing as clinical nurse leader
    differentiating your role from other leaders, 11–12
    elevator speech, 13
    portfolio, creation of, 13–15
    proposal
        development of CNL position, 9–10
        improvement of care and process, 6–9
        presentation of, 5
        purpose/mission, 5–6
Mayo Clinic, 130
McMaster University, 89
medical errors, 2, 54
Medicare, 82
Medicare Hospital Compare Data, 113
Medicare Provider Analysis and Review (MEDPAR), 113
medications
    instructions, 134
    management, 133–135
    shortages of, 40
MEDPAR. *See* Medicare Provider Analysis and Review
mentors, 10
    CNLs as, 91
    for dissemination, 176, 192
meta-analyses, 84
metrics that matter (MTM), 69
microsystem, 160
    cardiovascular surgery, 32–33
    culture, 54–55, 56
    level, disconfirmation at, 141
    needs, 26–27
    needs-based plan, 30–31
    patterns, 56, 69–70
    process improvement, 53–54
    processes, 56, 66–68
    professional nursing advocacy within, 163–165
    structure, 56, 63
Microsystem Academy Knowledge Center, 56, 70
microsystem assessment, 52, 70
    barriers to solving problems, 54–56
    in different settings, 56–70
    5P assessment, 26, 28–29, 56–70, 71–75
    ICU unit, reducing pressure ulcers in, 76–77
    problem identification, 53–54
    6S assessment, 26–27, 30
    state of microsystem meeting, 70, 76
mission statements, 57, 76
motivational interviewing, 130–131
MTM. *See* metrics that matter

National Academies of Medicine, 23
National Database of Nursing Quality, 113
national level advocacy, 169–171
National Quality Forum (NQF), 122, 123
navigation of healthcare system, 160–161
needs-based microsystem plan, 30–31
neighborhood, 132, 165
networking, 24–25

neurological units, inpatient, 66
new nurses, transition into CNL role, 18–19
NIGH. *See* Nightingale Initiative for Global Health
Nightingale, Florence, 80–81, 161, 171
Nightingale Initiative for Global Health (NIGH), 171
nonlinear systems, 38–39
nonverbal communication, 130
NQF. *See* National Quality Forum
nurse educators, 12
nursing advocacy. *See* professional nursing advocacy
nursing assistants, 66
nursing grand rounds, 178
nursing structure, assessment of, 18, 20

odds ratio (OR), 85
online video visits, 63
open-ended questions, 130, 133
OR. *See* odds ratio
organizational system
    complex adaptive systems, 41
    traditional systems, 41
organizational wellness programs, 162
organization(s)
    benefits to, 2
    collaboration with, 167
    conferences, 178–179
    culture, 169
    goals, 27
    needs, 27
    professional nursing advocacy within, 167–169
outcomes manager, CNL as, 7, 23, 161
outpatient care. *See* ambulatory care

p value, 85
Pareto charts, 108, 115–116
patient advocacy, 158
    fragmentation of care, 158–160
    navigation of healthcare system, 160–161
    wellness, promotion of, 161–162
patient-centered care, 81–82, 129–131, 132, 135
patient-centered medical homes (PCMHs), 23
PCMHs. *See* patient-centered medical homes
PCPs. *See* primary care providers
PDSA. *See* Plan, Do, Study, Act cycle
perioperative settings, 62, 63
pharmacists, 133
phone calls, follow-up, 131
PICOT question, 82–83
pictorial illustrations, 131
pill packs, 135
Plan, Do, Study, Act (PDSA) cycle, 25, 107
podium presentations, 189–191
population health, 23
portfolio, creation of, 13–15
poster presentations, 186–189, 190
poster-viewing sessions, 188–189
practice, clinical nurse leader, 17
    healthcare settings, 21–24
    infusion of CNL roles into, 27, 30–33
    role management, 24–27
    transitioning into CNL role, 18–20
presentations
    podium, 189–191
    poster, 186–189, 190
primary care, 36
    and organizational structure, 63
    patients, 61
    processes, 68
    professionals, 62–63
    purpose of, 57
    role of CNLs in, 23
primary care providers (PCPs), 124, 128, 133
primary data, 112
problem format, 191
process mapping, 68, 108
professional needs, 24–25

professional nursing advocacy, 162–163
  community level, 165–167
  within microsystem, 163–165
  national and global level, 169–171
  within organization, 167–169
Project Boost Model, 124
public health departments, 4
publications, 192–194
PubMed, 83

QI. *See* quality improvement
QSEN. *See* Quality and Safety Education for Nurses Institute
qualitative data, 112
qualitative research designs, 112
qualitative studies, 84
Quality and Safety Education for Nurses Institute (QSEN), 105
quality improvement (QI), 103, 104, 105, 169
  decreasing supply waste in surgical ICU, 117
  definition of, 105
  and EBP changes, 86
  failure mode and effects analysis, 110–111
  and financial savings, 115
  5 Why process, 110
  frameworks, 105–108
  project plan, 113, 114
  projects, 25
    data collection/analysis, 113–115
    research paper, 192–193
    root cause analysis, 109
  tools, 86, 115–117
quantitative data, 112
quantitative research designs, 112

randomized controlled trials, 84
rapport, building, 18, 20, 176
readmissions, hospital, 124, 125, 126–127
records, maintenance of, 14, 177

relationships
  CNL–manager, 54
  in healthcare system, 39–40
  leader–follower, development of, 45–46
  with patients, 61
  team, building, 19–20
reliability
  data, 113
  interrater, 114
  research articles, 85
research designs, 112
research study abstract, 182
retail clinics, 63
risk anticipator, CNL as, 9, 111
Rogers, Everett, 145, 146, 147, 150
role component-based intervention plan, 31–32
role modeling, 151, 159
root cause analysis, 108, 109
run charts, 116

salary of clinical nurse leaders, 25
sample of experimental studies, 85
SBAR (situation, background, assessment, recommendation) tool, 127
SDH. *See* social determinants of health
searching for evidence, 83–84
secondary data, 112
self-care, 162
self-management, 24–25
seven-step change theory (Lippett), 146, 147
shared decision-making, 130
short-term goals
  microsystem needs, 27
  professional needs, 25
sick nursing, 161
6S assessment, 26–27, 30
skilled nursing facilities (SNFs), 127, 128
SNFs. *See* skilled nursing facilities
social determinants of health (SDH), 61, 62, 132
Society of Hospitalists, 124

Squire 2.0 Guidelines, 192–193
staff
    acute care, 63, 66
    administrative, 54
    ambulatory care, 63
    following and supporting, 19
    frontline, 53, 61, 69, 150
    listening to, 19–20
    managerial, 53–54
    primary care, 62–63
    rapport with, 20, 53
    talking with, 21, 22, 53
statistical significance, 85
Stevens Star Model of Knowledge Transformation, 89
surveys, 112, 113–114
survival anxiety, 141
systematic reviews, 80, 84
systems analyst, CNL as, 9, 111
systems thinking, 40

TCM. *See* Transitional Care Model
teach-back techniques, 131
team approach for medication reconciliation, 133
team manager, CNL as, 9
team relationships, building, 19–20
telehealth, 162
telemedicine, 63
three-stage change model (Lewin), 145, 148
timeline, change project implementation, 151
title, 179–180
traditional leadership, 42–45
traditional systems
    vs. complex adaptive systems, 41
    leader characteristics in, 46

transactional leadership, 44
transdisciplinary teams, 55–56
transformational leadership, 44, 48
transition of care models, 124–125, 128
Transitional Care Model (TCM), 125
transitioning into CNL role
    experienced nurses, 20
    new nurses, 18–19
    team relationships, building, 19–20
transportation, 132
trust, building, 19

University of Pennsylvania, 125
unpredictability of healthcare system, 38
urgent care centers
    processes, 68
    professionals, 63
    purpose of, 58

VA. *See* Veterans Administration
validity
    data, 113–114
    research articles, 85
value-based purchasing, 104
Veterans Administration (VA), 3, 6
Virginia Office of Nursing Service, 87

wellness, promotion of, 161–162
WellStar Health System, 3–4
work action plan, 24
workers, healthcare, 42–45. *See also* staff

www.ingramcontent.com/pod-product-compliance
Lightning Source LLC
Chambersburg PA
CBHW061748030326
40576CB00012B/591